D0883420

Atlas of

FLUORESCEIN ANGIOGRAPHY

Atlas of

FLUORESCEIN ANGIOGRAPHY

Barbara A Harney PhD, FRCS, FRCOphth
Consultant Ophthalmologist
Royal United Hospital
Bath, UK

J Christopher Dean Hart BSc, MD, FRCS, FRCOphth
Consultant Ophthalmologist
Bristol Eye Hospital
Bristol, UK and
Honorary Professorial Fellow, Optometry
University of Wales
Cardiff, UK

Rodney H B Grey MA, FRCS, FRCOphth
Consultant Ophthalmologist
Bristol Eye Hospital
Bristol, UK

Photography and illustrations
Gill A Bennerson

M Wolfe

The *Slide Atlas of Fluorescein Angiography*, based on the contents of this book, is available. In the slide atlas format, the material is presented in a binder, together with numbered 35mm slides of each illustration. Further information is available from the publishers.

Copyright © 1994 Mosby–Year Book Europe Limited.
Published in 1994 by Wolfe Publishing, an imprint of Mosby–Year Book Europe Limited.

ISBN: 0–7234–1720–2

Printed in Spain by Grafos, S. A. Arte sobre papel

Cataloguing-in-Publication Data:
CIP catalogue records for this title from the British Library and US Library of Congress have been applied for.

For full details of all Mosby–Year Book Europe Limited titles, please write to Mosby–Year Book Europe Limited, Lynton House, 7–12 Tavistock Square, London WC1H 9LB, England.

PREFACE

Fluorescein angiography is an essential technique in the management of disorders of the fundus, yet many clinicians are uncertain about the indications for angiography and express a lack of confidence in their ability to interpret the results. We have drawn on our experience in providing a fluorescein angiographic service and teaching postgraduate students to write a practical book which we hope will answer many of the questions we are frequently asked.

Our experience is primarily in the field of fundus angiography using sequential photography, the technique employed in the majority of clinical departments, but in the final section we have included a brief account of other important techniques, some of which show great promise for the future.

This is an atlas with the emphasis on illustrations and the text is concise. We hope that the bibliography at the end of each chapter will be useful to those who would like more background information or detail.

ACKNOWLEDGEMENTS

Most of the photographs were drawn from the fluorescein library at Bristol Eye Hospital. We would like to thank all our colleagues from Bristol and from further afield who have referred patients for angiography and who have made efforts to fill gaps in our collection from their own libraries. We are very grateful to Professor D L Easty, Bristol Eye Hospital and Bristol University, and Dr P Meyer, of Adenbrooke's Hospital, Cambridge, for the benefit of their experience and their advice on the chapter on anterior segment angiography, and to Mr P Condon, Ardkeen Hospital, Waterford, Ireland, for his contribution to the section on sickle cell retinopathy. We should also mention Dr Ruth Raistrick, previously of Bristol Eye Hospital, who played an important part in building up the photographic library. We are particularly grateful to Mrs Gill Bennerson, Senior Ophthalmic Photographer, Bristol Eye Hospital, who was responsible for most of the photography and illustrations and who also contributed a great deal of time and moral support to the success of this project.

CONTENTS

1 Introduction

Over the thirty years since its introduction, fluorescein angiography has found a wide application in modern ophthalmology. Research groups and clinicians all over the world were quick to recognise its value, and there are few units in the developed world where this investigation is not readily available. The opportunity to study in detail the fine structure and dynamics of the ocular circulation has led to important advances in the understanding of many ocular diseases, and to changes in treatment.

Fluorescein dye has been used since the beginning of the century to study the retinal and choroidal circulation and fundus pathology. As early as 1910, Burk described his studies of human fundus pathology following the oral administration of fluorescein, while others investigated the ocular circulation of experimental animals. In the 1950s intravenous fluorescein was used clinically, but the results were not recorded photographically. The first fluorescein angiogram, in the cat, was produced by Flocks, Miller and Chao in 1959, and the first angiogram in humans was reported by Novotny and Alvis in 1961. Since then, the essentials of the technique have changed little. There have been advances in the design of cameras and the quality of the filters, but no substitute has been found for the dye itself.

Since the introduction of fluorescein angiography, indications for its use have changed. The understanding of certain fundus appearances through angiography has developed to the stage where the investigation is no longer necessary and is less often used. In other conditions, for example maculopathies associated with choroidal neovascularization and forms of retinal vascular occlusive disease, fluorescein angiography has become essential for determining management and monitoring treatment. This book concentrates on the current uses of fluorescein angiography in the management of disease. The role of fluorescein angiography as a research tool is mentioned only where this sheds light on its clinical use.

Valuable as this technique has proved to be, it should be regarded as an adjunct to, rather than a substitute for, clinical judgement. As with any investigation, but particularly with an invasive one with recognized complications, it is important that the use of angiography be limited to those cases where it is expected to make a positive contribution to management.

Bibliography

Alvis AL. Twenty-fifth anniversary of fluorescein angiography (letter). *Arch Ophthalmol* 1985;**103**:1269.

Blacharski PA. Twenty-five years of fluorescein angiography. *Arch Ophthalmol* 1985;**103**:1301–2

Burk A. Die klinische, physiologische und pathologische Bedeutung der Fluoreszenz im Auge nach Darreichung von Uranin. *Klin Mbl Augenheilk* 1910;**48**:445–54

Flocks M, Miller J, Chao P. Retinal circulation time with the aid of fundus cinephotography. *Am J Ophthalmol* 1959;**48**:3–6.

Maumenee AE. Doyne Memorial Lecture: Fluorescein angiography in the diagnosis and treatment of lesions of the ocular fundus. *Trans Ophthalmol Soc UK* 1968;**88**:529–56.

Novotny R, Alvis DL. A method of photographing fluorescence in circulating blood in the human retina. *Circulation* 1961;**24**:82–6.

2 Basics of angiography

Fluorescein dye

Fluorescein ($C_{20}H_{12}O_5$) is used in the form of its sodium salt, an orange-brown crystalline substance with a molecular weight of 376 (**1**). It belongs to the group of triphenylmethane dyes which includes fuchsin, gentian violet and eosin.

When exposed to light of a particular wavelength, fluorescent substances absorb energy and electrons are raised to a higher energy level. Energy is then spontaneously emitted in the form of light of a longer wavelength. Unlike phosphorescent substances, which continue to glow after excitation stops, light emission ceases when the stimulus is removed. When excited by blue light (465–490 nm), a sodium fluorescein solution emits yellow-green light (520–530 nm) (**2**).

The fluorescein molecule is small and diffuses freely out of all the body capillaries except those of the central nervous system, of which the retina is a part (see page 9). Between 80–90% of circulating dye is bound to plasma albumin; in this form it does not penetrate normal vascular walls, although the large fenestrations of the choriocapillaris allow the passage of some plasma proteins. Protein binding considerably reduces the level of light emitted, and it is the free dye which makes the most important contribution to clinically significant fluorescence. Fluorescence is further reduced by the absorption of exciting and emitted light by adjacent haemoglobin molecules.

Fluorescein is relatively pharmacologically inert. Dye is excreted by the liver and kidneys, some unchanged and some as the fluorescent metabolite, fluorescein monoglucuronide, and the non-fluorescent metabolites fluorescin and fluorescin glucuronide. The circulating fluorescein glucuronide is less fluorescent than fluorescein itself, but since it is bound to a lesser extent to plasma proteins it accounts for an increasing proportion of measured fluorescence with time after administration. Although not relevant to the interpretation of angiograms in the clinical setting, this factor may be important in studies of blood–ocular barrier kinetics.

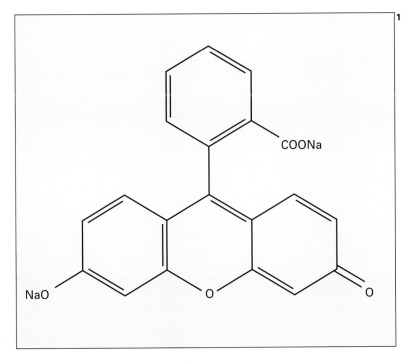

1 The sodium fluorescein molecule.

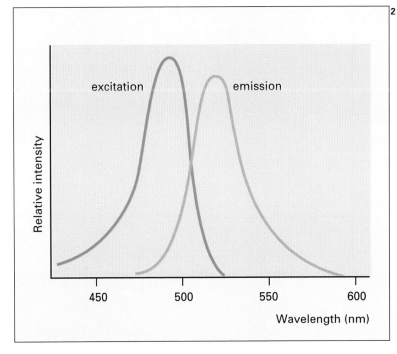

2 Excitation and emission spectra for fluorescein.

Photography

Following injection, a fundus camera is used to take sequential photographs through the dilated pupil. The passage of fluorescein through the retinal and choroidal vasculature is recorded on black and white film.

The camera incorporates an electronic flash unit with a xenon light source. An excitor filter allows only the transmission of blue light into the eye. Light returning from the fundus consists of reflected blue light as well as the yellow-green light emitted on stimulation of fluorescein dye. A barrier filter in the path of the beam returning to the camera eliminates the unwanted reflected blue light. In the early days of angiography, filters were less efficient, and there was a significant overlap between the range of wavelengths transmitted by the excitor and barrier filters (3). The green barrier filter used by Novotny and Alvis, for example, permitted approximately 5% transmission in the blue range, and their photographs had a visible background irrespective of fluorescence. Since then, the specificity of filters has improved, particularly with the introduction of interference filters, and pseudofluorescence due to transmitted reflected light is much reduced.

Other advances in light sources, recharging time, film quality and development techniques have also improved the quality of angiograms. Exposure time is reduced to milliseconds, thus reducing the effect of patient movement, and photographs are taken usually at 1–2 second intervals, compared with the 12 seconds to which Novotny and Alvis were restricted. Some cameras now enable the operator to select the area of fundus photographed (a range of 30–60°) and automatically record the time of each frame after injection. Advances not yet in routine use are described in Chapter 11.

Valuable information about differences in retinal thickness and the level of abnormalities can be obtained by stereophotography. Some cameras are fitted with stereo separators, but these are not essential in everyday clinical practice. It is possible to take paired stereophotographs where necessary by moving the camera beam manually from one side of the pupil to the other between exposures. The adjacent frames can then be studied using a pair of +10 to +15D spectacles to magnify and fuse the images.

There are a variety of films and processing techniques in use depending on local facilities, availability of materials, camera characteristics and departmental traditions.

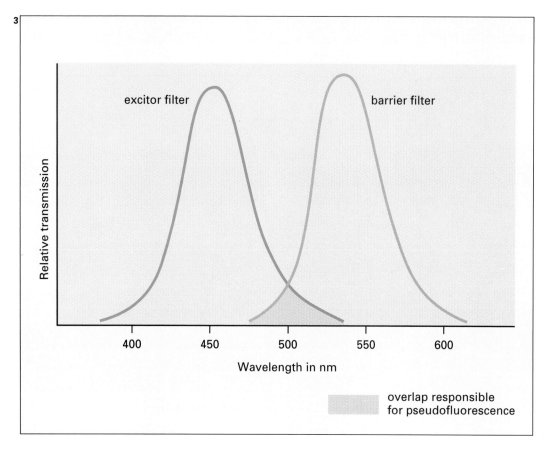

3 Diagram to illustrate pseudofluorescence.

The technique

Fluorescein is usually given intravenously. It is possible to give it orally, and under certain circumstances this can give useful information where there is extensive persistent hyperfluorescence as, for example, in the investigation of cystoid macular oedema, disc swelling or central serous chorioretinopathy. However, early details of the retinal circulation are not obtained and a significant number of angiograms may show no useful fluorescence at all. It may be the only acceptable route for a small child, or for an adult with difficult veins or a great fear of injections. It is argued, on the basis of comparison with other potential allergens, that the oral route is likely to be safer, but adverse reactions both mild and life threatening have been reported after oral administration.

The intravenous route is recommended wherever possible. The dye is used in concentrations of 10–25%. Satisfactory results are reported with all these concentrations and there does not seem to be any increase in adverse effects with increased concentrations. We use 3–5ml of a 20% solution.

It is very important that the patient receives a full explanation of the test. This should be given at the time the test is arranged. Patients are often very anxious, even if they do not articulate their fears, and there are a few common misconceptions. It is surprising, for example, how many people think that the dye will be injected directly into their eye. Some think that they are undergoing a treatment rather than an investigation, and some believe that they are going to be subjected to X-rays. Patients should be warned that their skin will be stained by the dye and that their urine will be a bright yellow. This is particularly important in the case of diabetics who should be specifically warned that the colour change may interfere with their urine testing. We also warn patients about the possibility of nausea as this can be quite alarming to the unprepared. It is convenient to include these explanations on a leaflet which is given to the patient when the appointment is made (**4**).

Pupils are dilated with topical tropicamide 1% and phenylephrine 10%. The patient is then seated comfortably at the camera. Initially, colour photographs are taken. These are necessary for later interpretation of the angiogram. A large vein is found in the antecubital fossa and clothing around the upper arm is loosened to ensure that the flow of dye is not impeded. Fluorescein solution is then injected quickly using a needle or an intravenous cannula (**5**). Care is taken to ensure that the needle is in the vein to avoid extravasation of dye into the subcutaneous tissues. Photographs are then taken at intervals of 1–2 seconds, starting immediately after injection, to ensure that the arrival of the dye and its transit through the choroidal and retinal circulation are recorded. At the end of the transit or 'run', photographs are taken of the fellow eye. Residual or 'late' photographs are taken after 2–5 minutes, or later if required.

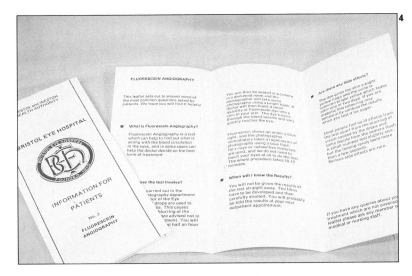

4 Explanatory leaflet used at Bristol Eye Hospital.

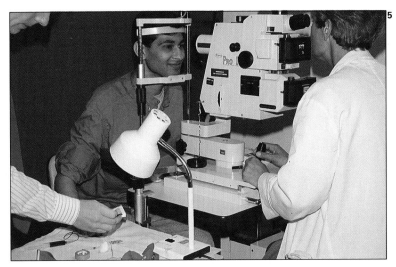

5 Fluorescein angiogram in progress.

Adverse effects and precautions

Although fluorescein angiography is relatively safe, there are recognized adverse effects. These are mostly mild, but some are more serious with well substantiated reports of fluorescein-related deaths (6).

There is evidence that in some cases problems have been caused by contaminants, but although the purity of the dye and quality control have improved reports of adverse reactions continue, suggesting that in a significant proportion of cases the dye itself is to blame.

Mild adverse reactions

Nausea and vomiting Nausea, sometimes accompanied by vomiting, is common with a reported incidence of 4–20%. It occurs quite suddenly within 20–30 seconds of the injection and, in the majority of cases, subsides within 2–3 minutes. Often the symptom is merely unpleasant, and elicited only on direct questioning. The early pictures have usually been obtained before nausea occurs, but if the patient is severely affected there may be delay in obtaining late transit photographs. Not all patients who have suffered nausea and vomiting experience these symptoms on subsequent occasions, but if this proves to be a problem, prophylactic antihistamines or anti-emetics such as metoclopramide are helpful.

Extravasation Extravasation of fluorescein implies poor technique and it should happen only rarely if appropriate checks are made before the dye is injected. Injection of fluorescein outside the vein is painful and should therefore be recognized early and the needle resited. The pain may last from a few minutes to several days and, if the problem goes unnoticed and insufficient dye reaches the circulation to give a good picture, the patient is faced with a further angiogram. There have been reports of skin necrosis following fluorescein extravasation requiring eventual skin grafting, but fortunately this is rare and probably represents an idiosyncratic reaction.

Intra-arterial injection This is an uncommon complication and can be avoided by feeling for pulsation before cannulating the vessel, and by observing the flow of bright red, oxygenated blood back into the syringe or tubing. If fluorescein is injected into an artery, the lower arm becomes an intense yellow colour and the patient notices sudden pain. Serious long-term sequelae have not been reported. First-aid treatment involves pressure over the injection site to avoid a haematoma.

Other minor effects Patients occasionally complain of paraesthesiae of tongue and lips, pruritus or dizziness. Fainting may occur, possibly associated more with the stress of the procedure than the dye itself. Urticaria may develop soon after the injection, or be noticed up to a few hours later. Patients with these less common symptoms should be watched carefully for at least an hour after injection in case they develop a more serious reaction.

Serious adverse reactions

It is the clinician's responsibility to ensure that the investigation is necessary and that those administering the dye are prepared to deal with any emergency that may arise.

Frequency Serious adverse reactions are rare, with figures ranging from 0·05–1·14%, depending on the definition of 'serious'. Life-threatening reactions are very rare, with an incidence probably less than 1 in 2000 (0·05%). However, there is no doubt that fatalities have occurred, with an estimated risk of death varying between 1 in 50 000 and 1 in 222 000. The discrepancy between these figures reflects the rarity of the event.

Adverse reactions			
mild	**allergic**	**cardiovascular**	**other**
yellow staining of skin and urine	urticaria	syncope	skin necrosis
nausea and vomiting	bronchospasm	myocardial infarction	lymphangitis
pain (associated with extravasation)	angioedema	cardiac arrhythmias	epileptiform seizure
feelings of faintness	anaphylactic shock	pulmonary oedema	carpo-pedal spasm
paraesthesiae		cerebral ischaemic event	

6 Adverse reactions.

Allergic reactions Serious reactions similar to those associated with acute hypersensitivity, and thus termed 'allergic', usually occur within minutes of injection and require emergency treatment. Acute bronchospasm, angioedema and anaphylactic shock have all been reported. Rapid treatment with adrenaline followed by appropriate specific treatment as required may be life-saving (**7**). Staff should be fully trained in emergency procedures and the necessary drugs and equipment readily at hand.

Patients with milder allergic responses, such as urticaria, are treated with oral or intramuscular antihistamines and need to be kept under observation for an hour or so in case a more serious reaction develops.

The nature of the 'allergic' reaction is not understood. Most of those affected have had no known previous exposure to the dye, except possibly in the form of eye drops. Although it is wise to be vigilant in patients with a previous history of allergy or asthma, serious reactions can occur in patients with no such history. Most serious allergic reactions develop usually within minutes of the injection and are rare after about 20 minutes.

Cardiovascular reactions A full range of cardiovascular events, from simple syncope to fatal myocardial infarction, have been reported in patients soon after angiography. Syncope is reported following 0·2–0·3% of angiograms. Although it is difficult to estimate the risk of more serious cardiac reactions – the events are very rare and reviews of complications have often been retrospective and have used different classifications – estimates from 1 in 4400 to 1 in 37 000 have been quoted. The cause of these complications is unknown. In some cases there may have been an 'allergic' basis for the cardiovascular collapse. In others, the stress of the investigation coupled with anxiety over the ocular condition may have precipitated the event in a susceptible patient. The instillation of phenylephrine eye drops could also be a contributing factor. The attending clinician and support staff should be fully conversant with cardiopulmonary resuscitation, and have the appropriate equipment and drugs at hand. A patient's cardiac condition should be taken into consideration when contemplating angiography. If the investigation is considered justifiable in the presence of significant cardiovascular disease, the patient requires observation for at least one hour after the angiogram.

Contraindications to fluorescein angiography

The only absolute contraindication to fluorescein angiography is a previous serious reaction to fluorescein. However, there are a number of relative contraindications:

- Previous mild reaction to fluorescein.
- Moderate to severe asthma with poor control.
- Recent stroke, myocardial infarction or unstable angina.
- Pregnancy. There is no evidence that fluorescein harms the fetus, but it is good practice to avoid any unnecessary medications during pregnancy.
- Lactation. Fluorescein is excreted in the breast milk and the baby would thus receive a dose of oral fluorescein. This can be avoided by expressing and discarding the milk following the test.

Renal dizease and renal dialysis are not generally considered to be a contraindication.

Care needs to be taken in patients with impaired lymphatic drainage, e.g. following radical mastectomy. The injection should be given into the unaffected arm to avoid lymphangitis and cellulitis.

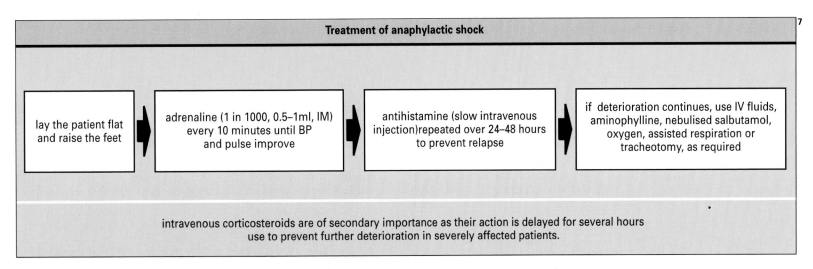

Treatment of anaphylactic shock 7

| lay the patient flat and raise the feet | ➤ | adrenaline (1 in 1000, 0.5–1ml, IM) every 10 minutes until BP and pulse improve | ➤ | antihistamine (slow intravenous injection)repeated over 24–48 hours to prevent relapse | ➤ | if deterioration continues, use IV fluids, aminophylline, nebulised salbutamol, oxygen, assisted respiration or tracheotomy, as required |

intravenous corticosteroids are of secondary importance as their action is delayed for several hours use to prevent further deterioration in severely affected patients.

7 Anaphylactic shock requires prompt, energetic treatment of laryngeal oedema, bronchospasm and hypotension.

Interference with laboratory tests

There are reports that fluorescein angiography can interfere with a range of laboratory tests, particularly those where a colorimetric method is used. Different processes and equipment may be affected to varying degrees, but the topic has not been comprehensively researched.

In the absence of more detailed information, it is recommended that blood for such investigations be taken before angiography or on the following day.

Bibliography

Bloom JN, Herman DC, Elin RJ *et al*. Intravenous fluorescein interference with clinical laboratory tests. *Am J Ophthalmol* 1989;**108**:375–9.

Bloome MA. Fluorescein Angiography: Risks. *Vis Res* 1980;**20**:1083–97.

Brown RE, Sabates R, Drew SJ. Metoclopramide as prophylaxis for nausea and vomiting induced by fluorescein. *Arch Ophthalmol* 1987;**105**:658–9.

Chahal PS, Neal MJ, Kohner EM. Metabolism of fluorescein after intravenous administration. *Invest Ophthalmol Vis Sci* 1985;**26**:764–8.

Grotte D, Mattox V, Brubaker R. Fluorescent, physiological and pharmacokinetic properties of fluorescein glucuronide. *Exp Eye Res* 1985;**40**:23–33.

Halperin LS, Olk RJ, Soubrane G, Coscas G. Safety of fluorescein angiography during pregnancy. *Am J Ophthalmol* 1990;**109**:563–6.

Jaanus SD. Dyes. Chapter 12. In: Bartlett JD, Jaanus SD, eds. *Clinical Ocular Pharmacology* 2nd Ed. Oxford: Butterworths, 1989: 323–35.

Jacob JSH, Rosen ES, Young E. Report on the presence of a toxic substance, dimethylformamide, in sodium fluorescein used for fluorescein angiography. *Br J Ophthalmol* 1982;**66**:567–8.

Karhunen U, Raitta C, Kala R. Adverse reactions to fluorescein angiography. *Acta Ophthalmologica* 1986;**64**:282–6.

Kinsella FP, Mooney DJ. Anaphylaxis following oral fluorescein angiography (letter). *Am J Ophthalmol* 1988;**106**:745.

Mattern J, Mayer PR. Excretion of fluorescein into breast milk (letter). *Am J Ophthalmol* 1990;**109**:598–9.

Nagataki S, Matsunaga I. Binding of fluorescein monoglucuronide to human serum albumin. *Invest Ophthalmol Vis Sci* 1985;**26**:1175–8.

Pacurariu RI. Low incidence of side effects following intravenous fluorescein angiography. *Ann Ophthalmol* 1982;**14**:32–6.

Stein MR, Parker CW. Reactions following intravenous fluorescein. *Am J Ophthalmol* 1971;**72**:861–8.

Watson AP, Rosen ES. Oral fluorescein: reassessment of its relative safety and evaluation of optimum conditions with use of capsules. *Br J Ophthalmol* 1990;**74**:458–61.

Yannuzzi LA, Rohrer KT, Tindel LJ *et al*. Fluorescein angiography complications survey. *Ophthalmology* 1986;**93**:611–17.

Zografos L. Enquête internationale sur l'incidence des accidents graves ou fatals pouvant survenir lors d'une angiographie fluoresceinique. *J Fr Ophtalmol* 1983;**6,5**:495–506.

3 Fundamentals of interpretation

A knowledge of certain aspects of the anatomy and physiology of the eye is important for the interpretation of fluorescein angiograms. Two independent factors have to be considered: the distribution of the dye within the ocular tissues, and the visibility of the dye.

The former depends on the structure of the blood vessels and the retinal pigment epithelium, and the affinity of the dye for the tissues. The latter depends on the concentration of the dye, the relative opacity of the optic media and camera characteristics.

The retinal circulation

The retinal blood vessels are derived from the central retinal artery, a branch of the ophthalmic artery. The main vessels pass outwards from the optic nerve head, branching to form a complex and variable pattern. These lie within the ganglion cell and nerve fibre layers, sometimes only separated from the inner limiting membrane by thin glial processes. The capillary beds are found in the nerve fibre and ganglion cell layers, and in the inner nuclear layer. There is a further network of radial peripapillary capillaries in the most superficial nerve fibre layer, which follows the pattern of the arcuate nerve fibres from the disc. There are no capillaries immediately adjacent to the larger vessels, and there is a capillary-free zone 400–500 μm in diameter at the fovea. The endothelial cells of retinal capillaries, like those elsewhere in the central nervous system, have tight junctions which prevent the passage of fluid between the cells.

In approximately 30% of eyes there is a cilioretinal artery, arising from the temporal aspect of the disc and supplying variable areas of the peripapillary and macular retina. Cilioretinal arteries are separate from the retinal arterial system, and may remain patent in central retinal artery occlusion (see page 34). The capillaries of this system also have tight junctions.

The choroidal circulation

The choroid is a specialized, highly vascular tissue which supplies the nutritional needs of the retinal pigment epithelium, and the outer retina as far the outer plexiform layer. Choroidal blood flow is much greater than is required to supply the metabolic demands of the retina, and blood leaving through the vortex veins remains highly oxygenated. The choroid may also act as a heat regulator, protecting the temperature-sensitive photochemistry of the rods and cones.

The posterior choroid is supplied by the short posterior ciliary arteries which originate from the ophthalmic artery. The lateral long posterior ciliary artery which arises from a distal short posterior ciliary artery supplies a recurrent branch to the posterior pole. Recurrent arteries from the anterior segment contribute to the supply of the anterior choroid.

The arterioles branch and reduce in size until they terminate in a densely packed capillary layer, the choriocapillaris. The choriocapillaris consists of large, thin-walled capillaries with fenestrations which allow the passage of relatively large molecules, including some plasma proteins. Although there are regional variations in architecture, the choriocapillaris of the posterior choroid shows a lobular pattern. Each lobule is supplied by a central precapillary arteriole, which drains into peripheral postcapillary venules and eventually into the vortex veins.

Early studies, using neoprene latex casts, suggested that the choroid was highly anastomotic. However, there is now evidence from anatomical and clinical studies that the choroid is segmentally supplied at the level of both the larger and smaller vessels, and that ischaemic damage can occur. Triangular and trapezoidal areas supplied by short posterior ciliary arteries or their larger branches have been mapped out, and triangular choroidal filling defects have been detected in cases of suspected acute choroidal ischaemia. Occlusion of smaller vessels is thought to lead to focal or geographic infarcts. However, the system is not truly end-arterial. Anastomoses occur between adjacent capillary lobules, which may explain the frequent rapid recovery from acute choroidal ischaemia.

The blood–retinal barrier

The inner blood–retinal barrier

The endothelial cells lining the capillaries of the retina have tight junctions forming the inner blood–retinal barrier. All fluid and metabolic transfer is an active process across the endothelial cells.

The outer blood–retinal barrier

Between the choroid and the retina lies the retinal pigment epithelium. The hexagonal cells are arranged in a monolayer and are connected by a system of tight junctions (zonae occludentes) which do not allow the diffusion of even small molecules between cells. Selective transport of nutrients occurs from the extravascular space of the choriocapillaris across the specialized cells of the pigment epithelium; transport of water and waste occurs in the other direction. This system forms the outer blood–retinal barrier.

Passage of the dye

In most individuals, fluorescein enters the choroidal circulation slightly ahead of the retinal circulation. In the choroid, it passes from the larger vessels to the choriocapillaris and freely diffuses into the extravascular space. Passage occurs readily through Bruch's membrane but under normal circumstances dye cannot proceed further forward into the retina because of the pigment epithelial barrier. The concentration of dye in the vessels and extravascular space falls with recirculation of the blood, but some is retained as staining in Bruch's membrane, the sclera and the lamina cribrosa (8).

In the retina, fluorescein is retained within the retinal vessels including the capillaries and under normal circumstances does not pass into the neural layers.

Visibility of the dye

The healthy neuroretina is transparent. Assuming clear media, the retinal vasculature is clearly defined when filled with dye. The retinal pigment epithelium contains melanin which significantly reduces transmission of fluorescent light from the choroid. The degree of pigmentation and the pattern of distribution vary from individual to individual, but in most cases the choroid is seen only as a glow with its vascular detail obscured. There is an increase in density of pigment within the retinal pigment epithelial cells at the macula which, together with the luteal pigment in the retina, reduces transmitted choroidal fluorescence further in this region. Melanocytes are present within the choroidal stroma, and this factor also contributes to variation in background fluorescence.

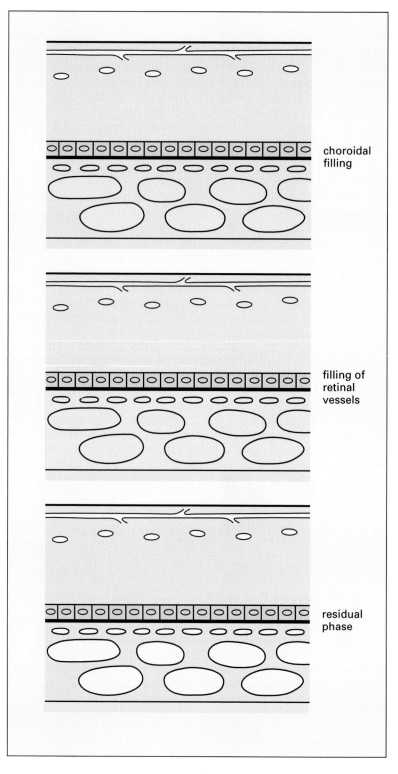

choroidal filling

filling of retinal vessels

residual phase

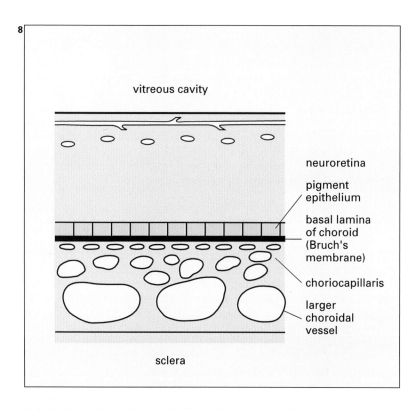

vitreous cavity

neuroretina

pigment epithelium

basal lamina of choroid (Bruch's membrane)

choriocapillaris

larger choroidal vessel

sclera

8 Left: The retina and choroid. Right: The passage of fluorescein dye through the eye. Filling of the choroid (top) and retinal vessels (middle), followed by the residual phase (bottom).

The normal angiogram

Dye appears in the eye about 10–15 seconds after injection into the antecubital vein. The time interval is variable and is affected by factors such as speed of injection, presence of constricting clothing around the arm, age and cardiovascular status. Dye usually first appears in the choroid and in a cilioretinal artery if present (**see 12**) followed within the next second by its appearance in the retinal arterioles. In practice, using sequential photography at 1–2 second intervals, it is rare to demonstrate purely choroidal fluorescence unless the retinal circulation is obstructed.

A normal fundus is shown in **9a**. The earliest fluorescence in this case is detected simultaneously in the retinal arterioles and the choroid (**9b**). The first faint glow appears 12 seconds after injection. The arterioles are faintly fluorescent. The incompletely filled arteriolar branches and the venules are seen as dark strands against the bright background, where they mask the underlying glow from the choroid. Fluorescein fills the arterioles (**9c**). The uneven appearance of the choroidal fluorescence is within normal limits. The larger, well-

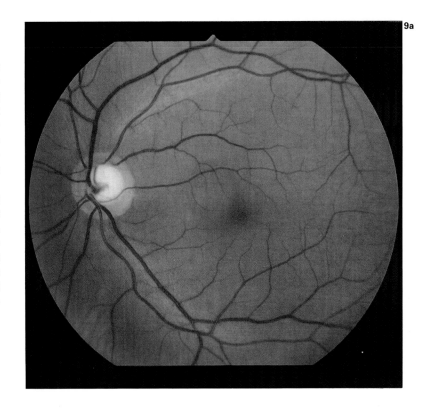

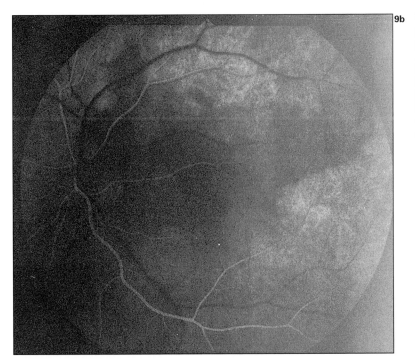
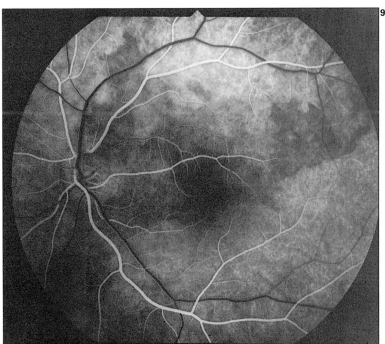

9(a–c) The healthy eye. **(a)** A normal fundus. **(b)** Early fluorescence 12 seconds after injection. **(c)** Fluorescein beginning to fill the arterioles.

defined patches are due to uneven filling of choroidal lobules and disappear within a few frames. Finer, persistent irregularities are due to variations in pigment density in the retinal pigment epithelium. Dye in choroidal vessels, in the extravascular space of the choroid and sclera and in Bruch's membrane all contribute to the background glow which persists throughout the angiogram. The macular area remains dark, as the underlying choroidal fluorescence is masked by the density of pigment in the pigment epithelium and by luteal pigment.

After 15 seconds, the fluorescein is just beginning to fill the veins from the small tributaries, outlining them on either side in a characteristic laminar pattern. The central column of blood arriving from the periphery has not yet become fluorescent (**9d**). The dye gradually fills the veins with a trilaminar appearance in places (**9e, 9f**). At peak fluorescence the frame appears very bright, as dye fills arterioles and veins. The laminar appearance of the veins is less obvious. Details of the macular capillary structure can be seen at this stage, but are usually more clearly delineated in earlier frames. There is a capillary-free zone (the foveal avascular zone) at the foveal centre (**9g, 9h**).

After 5 minutes the vessels are still hyperfluorescent, though less bright (**9i**). This is due to recirculating, diluted dye and not to staining of the vessel walls. Dye remains in the sclera and lamina cribrosa. Certain pathological conditions may become more apparent at this stage, where dye remains pooled in extravascular spaces. It is rarely necessary to wait more than 3–5 minutes after injection to demonstrate abnormal leakage. After about 20 minutes no dye is usually detectable angiographically in the normal eye.

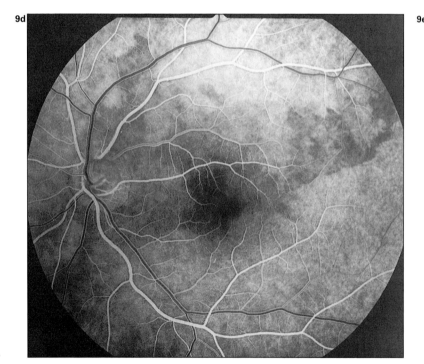
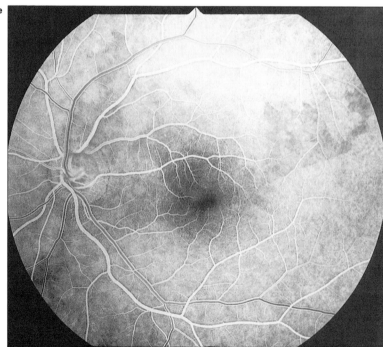

9 (contd) The healthy retina. **(d)** Fluorescence 15 seconds after injection. **(e)** Fluorescence 17 seconds after injection.

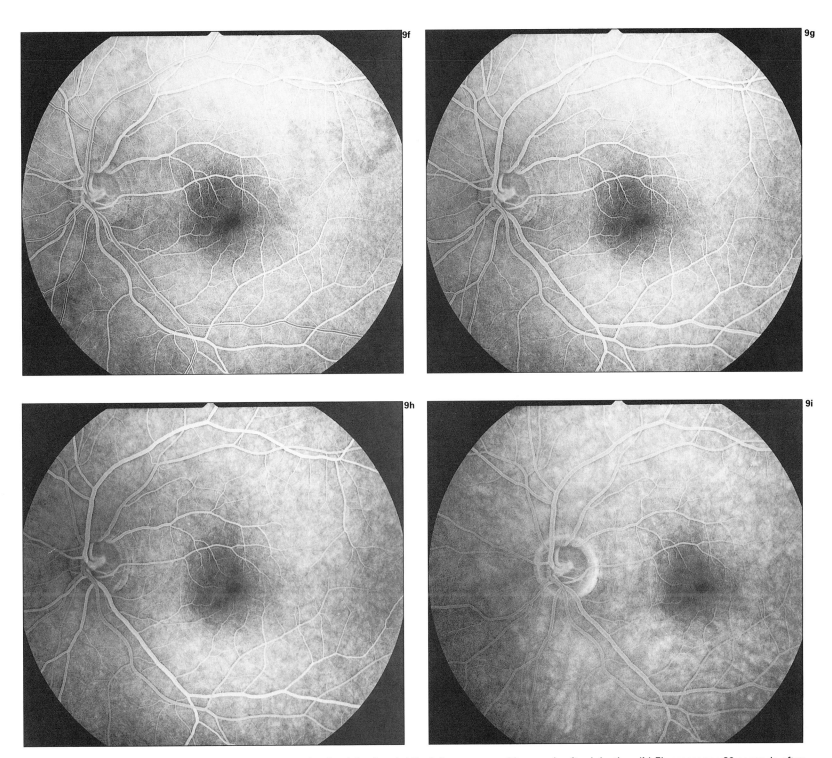

9 (contd) The healthy retina. **(f)** Fluorescence 18½ seconds after injection. **(g)** Peak fluorescence, 23 seconds after injection. **(h)** Fluorescence 30 seconds after injection. **(i)** Fluorescence 5 minutes after injection.

Principles of interpretation

Methods of examination

The angiogram can be examined as a negative, a positive transparency (contact sheet), or as a print. We routinely use negatives because quality is inevitably lost with every reproduction, and because preparation of contact sheets is costly and time consuming. With experience, it poses no problem to switch between negative and positive. Many methods of magnification are available. Perhaps the simplest and most convenient in the clinic setting is the 20D indirect ophthalmoscope lens against a light box. For more careful study, and to allow discussion or teaching, various projection systems are available. Adjacent frames taken to form stereo pairs are viewed through a pair of +10D spectacles.

A colour photograph should always be available for comparison with the angiogram when the findings are reported. Important ophthalmoscopic features which are not reliably reproduced on colour photographs (e.g. the presence of subretinal fluid) should be noted when the patient is examined before angiography. Occasionally, particularly when the colour photographs are of poor quality, adequate assessment of the angiograms requires re-examination of the patient.

Variants of normal

The key to the interpretation of the abnormal is a thorough understanding of the range of normal appearances. Patchy choroidal filling and irregularities in pigmentation leading to irregular fluorescence have already been mentioned. Pigmentation varies with skin and hair colour, resulting sometimes in quite marked differences in the amount of transmitted choroidal hyperfluorescence (**10,11**). Retinal vascular patterns vary (**12**), as do sizes, shapes and fluorescent patterns of optic discs. Pigment around the disc does not usually pose a problem, but subtle scleral rings may not be noticed on clinical examination, and the associated hyperfluorescence may be misinterpreted as a pathological finding.

Sometimes artefacts caused by defects or dirt within the optics of the camera, or by problems in processing, simulate abnormalities (**13**)—it is not unknown for such a 'lesion' to be presented at a clinical meeting! Scrutiny of adjacent frames should readily demonstrate that the abnormality occurs at different positions relative to the anatomical landmarks.

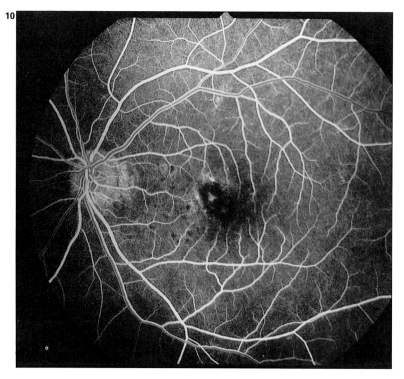

10 An angiogram was performed on a man of Chinese origin to investigate a macular lesion. The reduction of background choroidal fluorescence associated with greater fundus pigmentation is in marked contrast to the fluorescence illustrated in **9** (compare with **9e**).

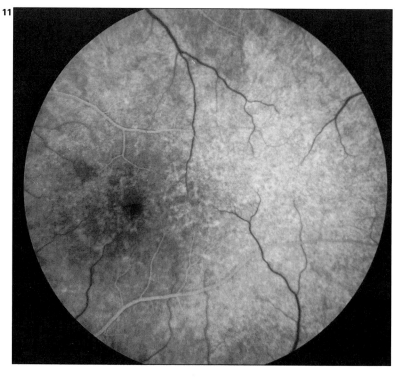

11 An angiogram of an albinoid fundus showing increased transmission of choroidal fluorescence, with marked background fluorescence already visible in this early frame.

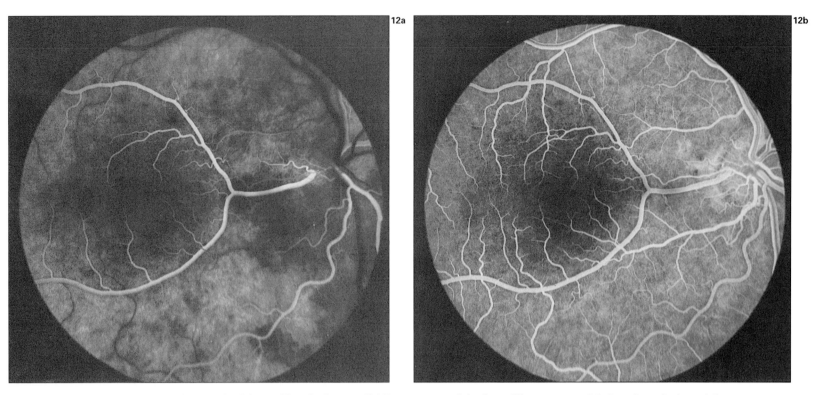

12 An unusual vascular pattern at the macula. A large cilioretinal artery dividing to surround the fovea fills, as expected, before the retinal arterioles.

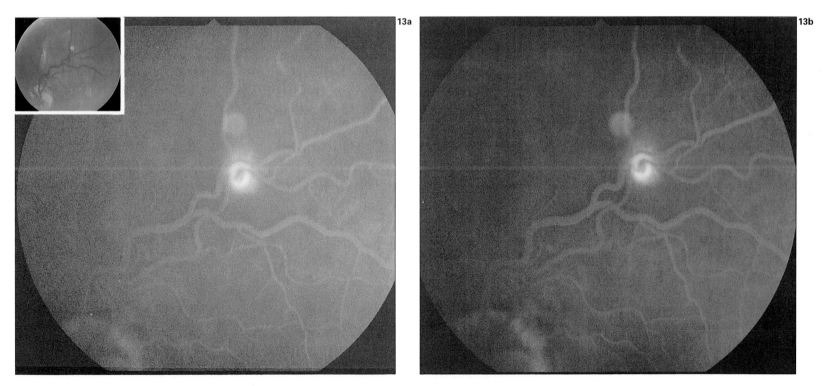

13 Late photographs showing persistent hyperfluorescence from a leaking retinal macroaneurysm. In **a**, there appears to be a lesion of similar size above it. Examination of an adjacent frame (**b**) shows that the relative position of the upper lesion has changed, suggesting that it is an artefact. The colour photograph (inset) also demonstrates the artefact.

The interpretation of abnormalities

The demonstration of fluorescence on an angiogram depends on the presence of the dye within the tissues, as well as on the transmission of the exciting blue light and the emitted yellow light through the optic media. Pathological hyperfluorescence is a result of either abnormal accumulation of dye where it is not normally found, or of increased transmission of emitted light through defects in the pigmented structures through which it passes. The main example of the latter is the increased fluorescence observed from the choriocapillaris following loss of melanin in the pigment epithelium. Pathological hypofluorescence is the result of absence of dye where it would normally be expected, or of the blocking of light transmission by opaque structures or deposits.

Autofluorescence occurs in the absence of fluorescein. Certain structures are inherently fluorescent and are demonstrated photographically before the dye is injected. Exposed optic nerve drusen are the classic example and a pre-injection photograph sometimes provides the diagnosis (**14**, also see p. 113). Pseudofluorescence is due to reflected light from the eye passing through the camera filters with exposure of the film and a misleading impression of fluorescence. Good quality exciting filters with little overlap in their transmission properties minimize this problem, but large areas of exposed sclera can sometimes lead to marked pseudofluorescence.

Hyperfluorescence

There are a number of causes of hyperfluorescence (**15**).

Leakage This is a term which is often misused in the context of fluorescein angiography. Sometimes it is used synonymously with hyperfluorescence whatever the cause, leading to misunderstanding and misinterpretation. Leakage implies permeability of blood retinal barriers and may be focal or diffuse. It is characterized by the spread of hyperfluorescence with indistinct boundaries (**16**).

Pooling Dye collecting in fluid-filled spaces leads to characteristic patterns on angiography. In a pigment epithelial detachment, fluid collects under the pigment epithelium and gradually becomes hyperfluorescent during the course of the angiogram (**17**). The lesion fills with variable speed and there may be irregularities in its margins and in the intensity of fluorescence, but there is a characteristic homogeneous appearance to the fluorescence and the boundaries of the lesion remain unchanged during the course of the angiogram. In central serous retinopathy (**18**; see also p. 80), dye appears in a fluid space between the retinal pigment epithelium and the neuroretina, giving a picture of spreading hyperfluorescence. In cystoid macular oedema the dye collects within cystic spaces in the neuroretina (**19**; see also p. 53). These conditions will be discussed in greater depth in Chapters 4–10.

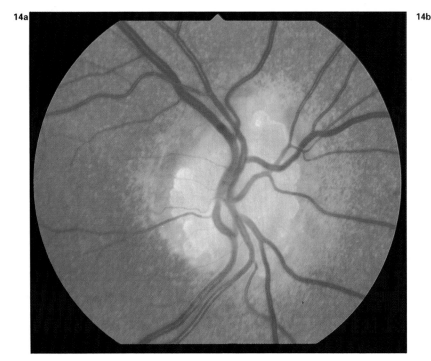

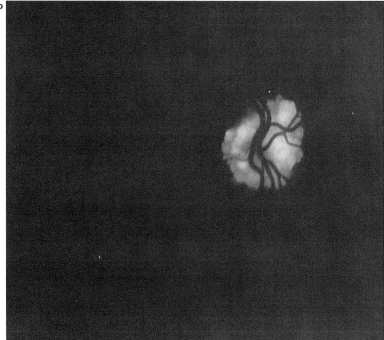

14 A photograph taken using the excitor filter before the injection of dye to demonstrate the autofluorescence of drusen of the optic nerve head. The angiogram of the fellow eye is illustrated in **104**.

accumulation of dye (hyperpermeability)	leakage across blood–retinal barrier	inner	microaneurysms retinal new vessels
		outer	choroidal new vessel network
	pooling in fluid spaces		central serous retinopathy pigment epithelial detachment cystoid macular oedema
	staining	normal	disc sclera
		abnormal	drusen vessel walls in ischaemia scar tissue
increased transmission		normal	hypopigmentation of retinal pigment epithelium
		abnormal	retinal pigment epithelial atrophy

15 Manifestations of hyperfluorescence.

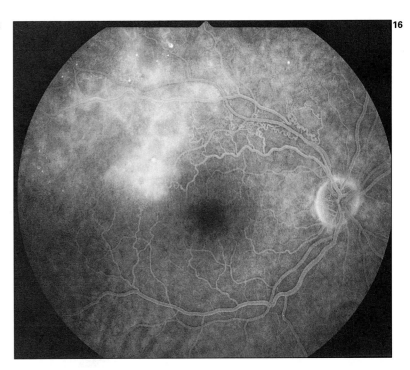

16 Leakage. A late photograph demonstrating leakage from damaged retinal vessels following branch vein occlusion.

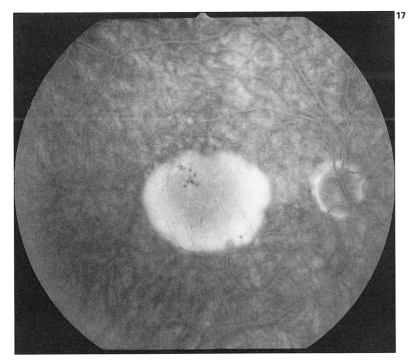

17 Pooling. A pigment epithelial detachment.

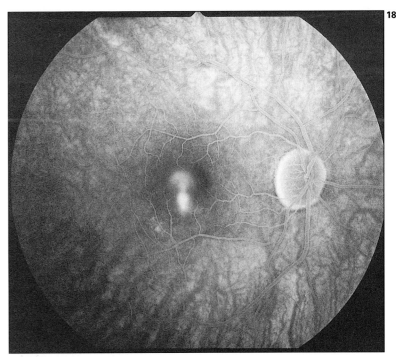

18 Pooling. A late picture demonstrating hyperfluorescence in central serous retinopathy.

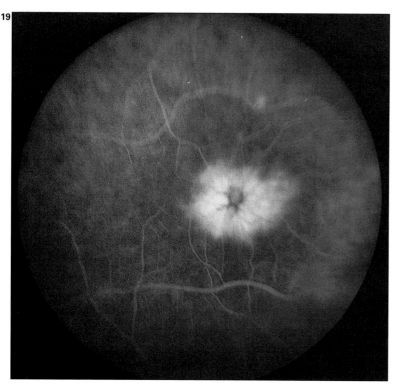

19 Pooling. A late picture showing the pattern of hyperfluorescence in cystoid macular oedema. The patient had undergone intra-capsular cataract extraction.

Staining This is a term which is often confused with leakage. It should be reserved for those situations where dye is taken up and retained by tissues after it has left the ocular circulation. Normal structures which retain dye are the sclera, the lamina cribrosa and Bruch's membrane.

Staining accounts for the late fluorescence of the normal optic disc and the hyperfluorescence of the underlying sclera exposed after a choroidal rupture or in cases of chorioretinal atrophy (**20**). Certain types of drusen retain dye and remain hyperfluorescent into the late stages of the angiogram. Staining of vessel walls may be seen in vasculitis and in areas of retinal ischaemia, and staining of scar tissue is observed in conditions such as advanced disciform age-related maculopathy.

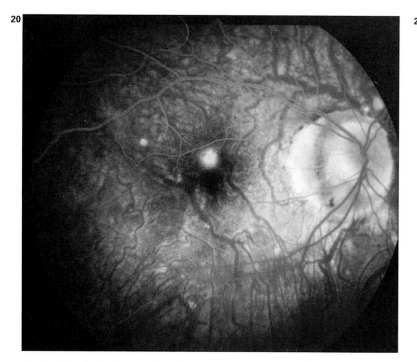

20 Staining. Late picture of a myopic fundus showing persistent fluorescence of the disc, and of the sclera exposed at the temporal disc margin. The patient has a small, discrete neovascular membrane at the fovea and the angiogram was performed to assess whether it would be amenable to treatment.

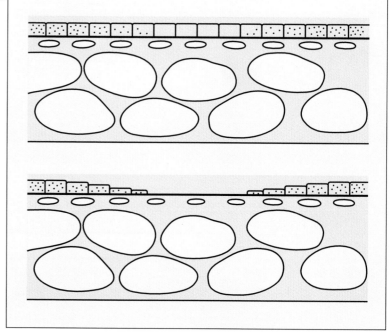

21 Diagram to illustrate a transmission or 'window' defect. Upper: Reduction of density of pigment in the pigment epithelium. Lower: Thinning of the pigment epithelium and choriocapillaris.

Transmission or 'window' defect (**21,22**) This is a common finding, especially in the older age group. Where there is reduction of pigmentation without a breach in the physiological barrier between the neuroretina and the choroidal extravascular space, the fluorescence of the underlying choroid is more clearly seen. The shape and size of the hyperfluorescent patch corresponds to the patch of atrophy seen on fundoscopy or photography and does not alter throughout the angiogram, although the degree of hyperfluorescence varies. Window defects become apparent early in the angiogram when the choroid fills, and then fade as it empties. They may remain detectable for longer in situations where the staining of the underlying sclera is exposed. Often the edges of the atrophic area are well-defined, but sometimes, where the defect blends into the surrounding normal area, leakage may be suspected. A careful study of subsequent frames will demonstrate the unchanging shape and size of the defect, and comparison with good-quality colour pictures is helpful.

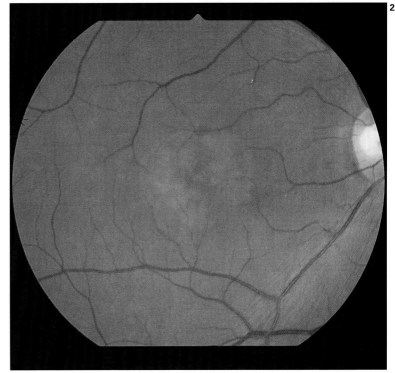

22a

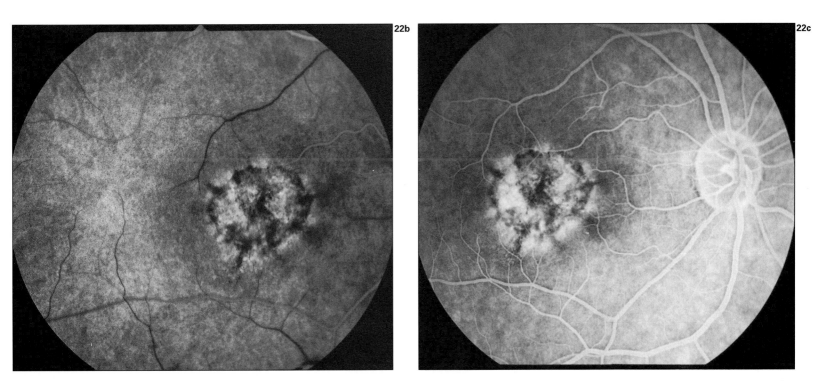

22b 22c

22 Window defect. **(a)** The macula of a young woman with symptoms suggesting a cone dystrophy. The other eye showed similar changes. **(b,c)** demonstrate the window defect corresponding to areas of the retinal pigment epithelial atrophy seen on colour photographs. The hyperfluorescence varies in intensity throughout the angiogram but the size and shape of the defects remain constant. The pattern of hypofluorescence corresponds to areas of pigmentation and represents masking.

Hypofluorescence

Hypofluorescence can have a number of causes (**23**).

Blockage or masking Optically opaque structures in the path of the light between the fundus and the camera cause hypofluorescence by masking. The normal retinal pigment epithelium provides a uniform barrier of melanin in front of the choroid which masks details of the choroidal circulation. Absence of this melanin in pathological states provides the explanation for window defects. Masking is usually the result of increased melanin deposition or the presence of haemorrhage, but may on occasion follow deposition of material within the pigment epithelium or neuroretina. Haemorrhage within the neuroretina leads to well-defined patches of uniform and profound hypofluorescence corresponding precisely to the area of extravasated blood. Such masking is readily distinguishable from the hypofluorescence resulting from a retinal filling defect, where the choroidal circulation is intact (**24**). More examples are given in Chapters 4–10.

Certain deposits in the fundus which are very apparent ophthalmoscopically may be almost invisible on angiography. Dense retinal exudates or Best's macular dystrophy (see **101**) may be unobserved on fluorescein angiography and are better recorded by colour or red-free photography.

23

masking of normal dye transit	media opacities	vitreous haemorrhage lens/corneal opacities
	pigment accumulation	**blood** preretinal intraretinal subretinal
		melanin retinal pigment epithelium choroid
	other	exudates oedema fluid } rarely
failure of dye circulation	retinal vessel closure	large vessel capillary
	choroidal vessel closure	segmental (large vessel) micro-infarcts optic nerve ischaemia

23 Causes of hypofluorescence.

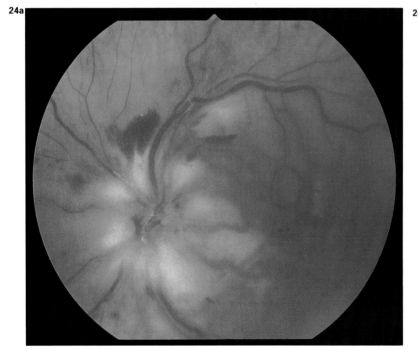

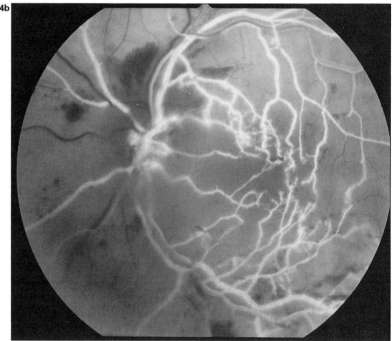

24 Masking, filling defect. This man presented with profound visual loss in one eye. (**a**) The fundus appearance. (**b**) A diagnosis of central retinal vein occlusion was made and an angiogram performed to assess the retinal circulation. Widespread nonperfusion was confirmed and no areas of capillary perfusion are present. The angiogram demonstrates the contrast between the masking due to retinal haemorrhage and the less profound hypofluorescence due to absence of dye within the retinal capillary bed.

Opacities in the cornea, lens and vitreous frequently degrade the picture by reducing and scattering fluorescence. Nuclear sclerosis absorbs large amounts of blue light causing poor excitation of fluorescein. However, there are occasions where, despite the presence of moderate opacification of the media, angiography can detect lesions not easily visible on fundoscopy: for example, in a patient with lens opacities.

Filling defects (see **24**) Hypofluorescence resulting from filling defects in the choroidal and retinal vasculature is usually distinguishable from that caused by masking by the shape and intensity of the hypofluorescent area, and by comparison with colour photographs. Hypofluorescence due to masking is profound and persists through the angiogram. It often corresponds in shape to an area of readily distinguishable pigmentation or haemorrhage detected on colour photographs. A filling defect, however, is often difficult to detect clinically.

Occlusion of the choroidal vasculature will lead to hypofluorescence in a segmental or lobular pattern, depending on the size of the vessel affected. The characteristic pattern will be seen only on the very early frames before fluorescein fills the extravascular space in the choroid. A pathological defect must be distinguished from the normal pattern of segmental choroidal filling.

Retinal filling defects range in size from small patches of capillary nonperfusion to complete sectors, and on occasions the entire retina.

The affected area is distinguishable from adjacent healthy retina by its relative hypofluorescence, and its uniform, featureless appearance. The intensity of the fluorescence varies with the fluorescence of the underlying structures.

Further examples of filling defects are given in Chapter 4.

Indications for angiography

Fluorescein angiography remains an essential investigation, and without ready access to this facility patient care is compromised. Indications can be summarized as follows:

- To make or confirm a diagnosis, e.g. differential diagnosis of pigmented choroidal lesions, exudative macular lesions, etc.
- To assess prognosis, e.g. estimation of macular nonperfusion in retinal vascular disease.
- To determine need for treatment, e.g. estimation of extent of retinal non-perfusion in central retinal vein occlusion, or assessment of size and position of subretinal neovascular network.
- To monitor the progress of disease, e.g. growth of a fundus tumour, or the effect of treatment, e.g. following laser photocoagulation of subretinal neovascularization, or medical or surgical treatment of cystoid macular oedema.

It is important that clinicians referring patients for angiography should be certain that the result of this invasive and potentially dangerous investigation will influence management.

Bibliography

Amalric P. Choroidal vascular ischaemia. *Eye* 1991;**5**:519–27.

Ernest JT. Macrocirculation and microcirculation of the retina. In: Ryan SJ *et al. Retina*. St Louis: Mosby, 1989: Chapter 7.

Ernest JT. Choroidal circulation. In: Ryan SJ *et al. Retina*. St Louis: Mosby, 1989: Chapter 8.

Foulds WS. The choroidal circulation and retinal metabolism – an overview. *Eye* 1990;**4**:243–8.

Gass JDM. *Stereoscopic atlas of macular diseases*. St Louis: Mosby, 1987: Chapters 1 (Normal macula) and 2 (Pathophysiologic and histopathologic bases for interpretation of fluorescein angiography).

Guyer DR, Schahat AP, Green WR. The choroid: structural considerations. In: Ryan SJ *et al. Retina*. St Louis: Mosby, 1989: Chapter 2.

Hayreh SS. Recent advances in fluorescein fundus angiography. *Br J Ophthalmol* 1974;**58**:391–412.

Hayreh SS. *In vivo* choroidal circulation and its watershed zones. *Eye* 1990;**4**:273–89.

Hurtes R. Evolution of ophthalmic photography. In: Justice J Jr. *Ophthalmic photography*. Town: Little, Brown and Co, 1982: Chapter 1.

Justice J Jr. *Ophthalmic photography*. New York: Little, Brown and Co, 1982: Chapters 2 (Ocular fundus photography) and 3 (Fluorescein angiography).

Olver JM. Functional anatomy of the choroidal circulation: methyl methacrylate casting of human choroid. *Eye* 1990;**4**:262–72.

Schatz H. Fluorescein angiography: basic principles and interpretation. In: Ryan SJ *et al. Retina*. St Louis: Mosby, 1989: Chapter 57.

Sigelman J, Ozanics V. Retina. In: Tasman W, Jaeger EA. *Duane's Foundations of Clinical Ophthalmology*. Philadelphia: JB Lippincott, 1990: Chapter 19.

Torczynski E. Choroid and suprachoroid. In: Tasman W, Jaeger EA. *Duane's Foundations of Clinical Ophthalmology*. Philadelphia: JB Lippincott, 1990: Chapter 22.

Wolff E. *Anatomy of the eye and orbit*. London: HK Lewis, 1976.

4 Retinal vascular disease

Retinal vascular disease is an important cause of visual loss. In Chapters 4–10 a range of conditions is described emphasising those encountered most frequently and the circumstances where angiography is of particular value.

Venous occlusion

Branch retinal vein occlusion

Branch retinal vein occlusion is a common cause of retinal vascular disease, particularly in hypertensive patients (25–29). Diagnosis is based on the recognition of the characteristic segmental distribution of intraretinal vascular changes and is seldom in doubt. The most striking feature of the acute phase is the retinal haemorrhages which are scattered over the affected sector. The occluded vein is dilated, and the site of obstruction at an arteriovenous crossing is often apparent (25,27). Preretinal oedema and cotton wool spots may be present. Over several months the haemorrhages gradually disappear, but oedema sometimes persists and exudates may develop. After resolution of the acute phase, signs of past occlusion include irregularities and dilatation of the microvasculature, sheathing of the venules, collateral vessels (29) and neovascularization of the disc or retina. The eventual outcome varies from complete functional recovery to severe visual loss. There are three main sight-threatening complications:

- Macular oedema.
- Macular nonperfusion.
- Neovascularisation leading to vitreous haemorrhage.

Indications for angiography

Angiography is rarely required for diagnosis in the acute phase. It is occasionally helpful in differentiating between a small macular branch vein occlusion, telangiectasis or a choroidal neovascular network in an elderly patient. In long-standing cases, where signs are minimal and the diagnosis uncertain, angiography sometimes demonstrates that a small patch of retinal vascular abnormality or oedema is the result of a past retinal vein occlusion.

Although unnecessary for diagnosis, fluorescein angiography is of great value in the management of branch vein occlusion in the following circumstances:

- to determine the precise cause of loss of visual acuity, differentiating between haemorrhage, oedema and macular ischaemia
- to assess the extent of retinal capillary closure
- to assess the degree of hyperpermeability of retinal vessels

Determining the cause of visual loss Visual recovery during the first 4–6 months after the acute event, as haemorrhage clears and oedema resolves, is dramatic in some cases. This is especially true where the perifoveal arcade has been preserved (compare 25,26). Angiography after resolution of central haemorrhages is useful for prognosis and the planning of any laser treatment if visual function remains compromised.

Assessment of retinal capillary closure The extent of retinal ischaemia has important prognostic significance (27,28,29). Widespread nonperfusion involving large areas of the peripheral retina is associated with a greater risk of retinal or optic disc neovascularization. Although at present prophylactic treatment is not recommended, an assessment of the area of ischaemia helps when planning the frequency of follow-up appointments and the date of final discharge. Once new vessels appear, scatter photocoagulation over the affected area promotes regression and reduces the risk of subsequent vitreous haemorrhage.

Small occlusions involving less than one quadrant rarely lead to neovascularization, even if considerable capillary closure is present; however, vein occlusions affecting a quadrant or more are often associated with large areas of nonperfusion and there is a real risk of subsequent neovascularization. It is difficult to be precise about the quantitative relationship between area of nonperfusion and risk of neovascularisation as different studies have used different criteria, but there is a high risk if the nonperfused areas are more than 5 disc diameters in size (28).

Assessment of hyperpermeability Macular oedema is caused by leakage of plasma from damaged capillaries (25). There may be associated deposition of exudate, or the formation of intraretinal cystoid spaces. Visual loss can occur even in the presence of apparently intact perifoveal capillaries with the spread of oedema and the deposition of exudate from more distal sites within the macular area. A proportion of patients show some recovery over time and it has been difficult to prove the benefits of laser treatment. Recent studies have suggested that treatment in selected cases may be beneficial, and in these cases fluorescein angiography is essential to confirm the presence and position of hyperpermeable vessels.

Central retinal vein occlusion

Central retinal vein occlusion is an important cause of visual loss (30–33). Diagnosis is based on the characteristic fundus appearance. In the acute phase, there is dilatation and tortuosity of the veins, swelling of the disc and varying amounts of retinal haemorrhage and oedema. Cotton wool spots are often present. As in branch vein occlusion, central vision is affected by retinal dysfunction caused by oedema or ischaemia.

Classifications of central retinal vein occlusion are confusing. Certain terms which have been used—*complete, incomplete, threatened, venous stasis*—imply an understanding of the pathological process in individual cases for which there is insufficient evidence, and are not helpful from the point of view of management. As in branch retinal vein occlusion, the extent of capillary nonperfusion determines the likelihood of neovascular complications. It is therefore more useful to describe the occlusion in terms of retinal perfusion and retinal capillary integrity. Fundus neovascularization is less common in central retinal vein occlusion than in ischaemic branch vein occlusion. However, neovascularisation of the iris and iridocorneal angle leading to neovascular glaucoma is a frequent and severe complication.

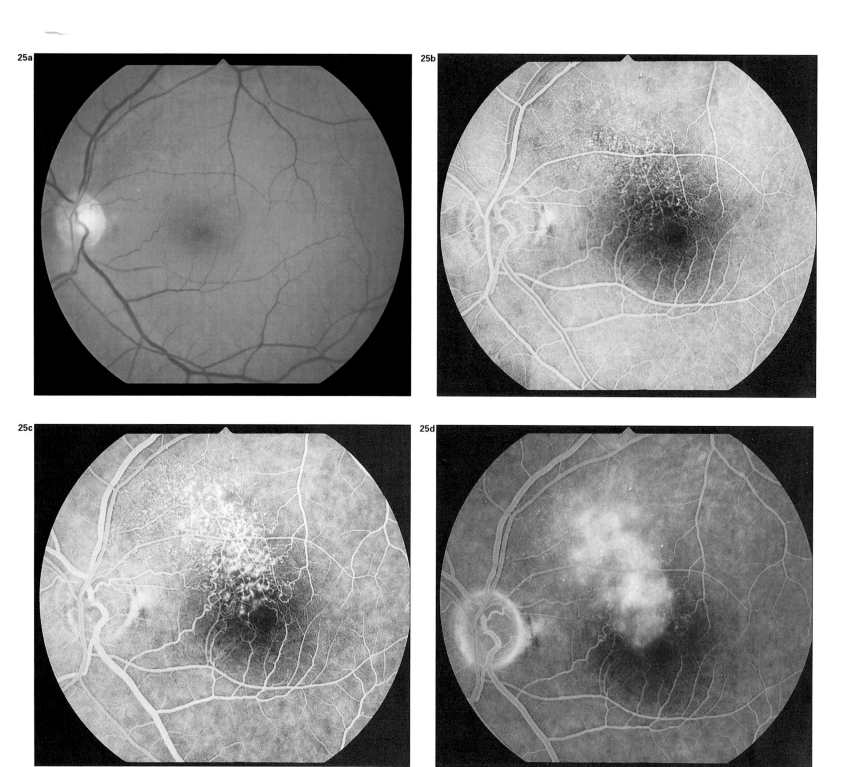

25 Branch retinal vein occlusion – hyperpermeability. A 53-year-old man noticed a rapid deterioration of vision in his left eye. His blood pressure was 170/105. The angiogram was performed a year later when the visual acuity had improved to 6/6. (**a**) The occlusion has occurred at a point where the superior temporal arteriole crosses a branch of the vein. (**b**) Surviving capillaries in the affected territory are dilated and tortuous, but with very little capillary closure. The parafoveal arcade is intact. (**c**) Increased hyperfluorescence from the damaged inner blood-retinal barrier. (**d**) Late phase showing diffuse intraretinal leakage.

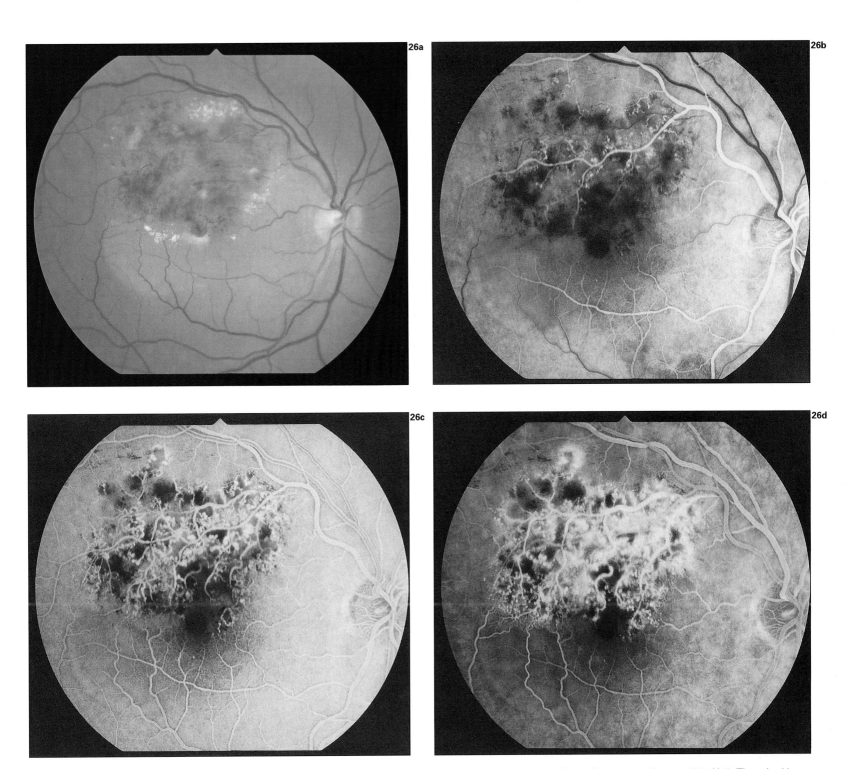

26 Branch retinal vein occlusion: foveal ischaemia. A 50-year-old man noticed deterioration in his right central vision. His visual acuity was 6/60, N48. There had been no improvement a year later. (**a**) Upper temporal branch vein occlusion with haemorrhage, oedema and an encircling ring of exudate. (**b,c,d**) Details of the capillary bed are partly obscured by haemorrhage. The visible capillaries over the affected area show dilatation and tortuosity with spreading hyperfluorescence, indicating leakage of dye. In spite of foveal haemorrhage, the angiogram shows that the upper part of the capillary ring at the edge of the capillary-free zone has been interrupted and there is closure of capillaries above the fovea.

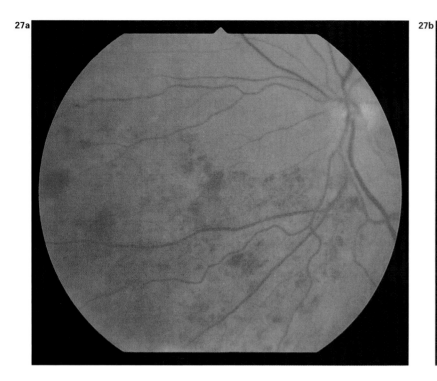

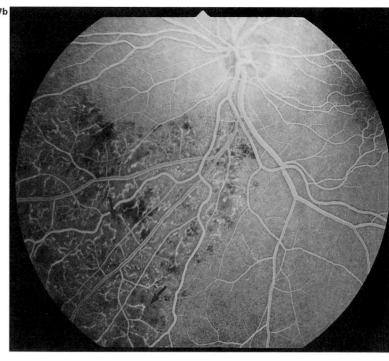

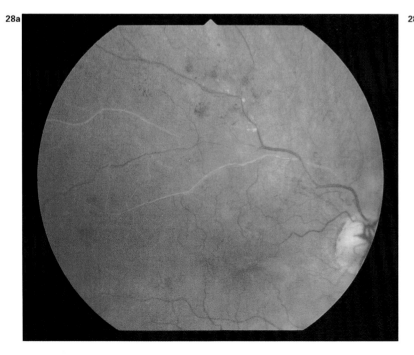

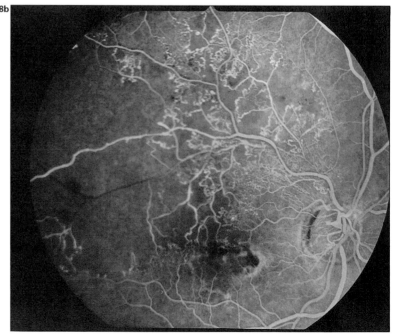

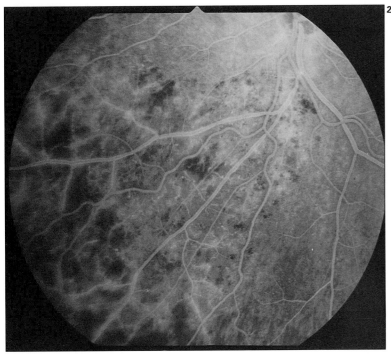

27 Branch retinal vein occlusion – mild/moderate nonperfusion. A 72-year-old woman was found to have reduced visual acuity in her left eye, VA 6/12. (a) Examination showed a cellophane maculopathy, but there was also evidence of a venous occlusion in the inferonasal quadrant. (b) The inferior nasal branch leaves a common trunk below the disc and is occluded soon after as it passes beneath the inferior temporal branch artery. A capillary bed is present over the most of the affected areas, but there are areas of closure (arrows) which appear to enlarge towards the periphery. Note the contrast between the dense hypofluorescence of the haemorrhages and the homogeneous grey hypofluorescence, representing capillary filling defects. (c) In the late picture, the walls of the affected vein and its larger branches are hyperfluorescent where they pass through ischaemic territory.

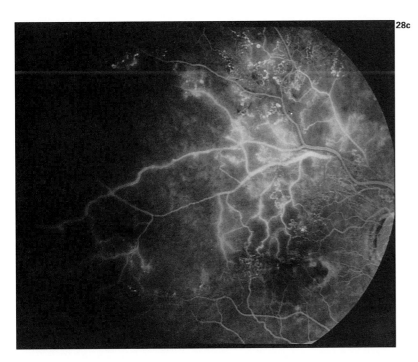

28 Branch retinal vein occlusion: severe ischaemia. A fit 55-year-old woman noticed a partial loss of vision in the lower field of her right eye. Over the following two weeks her vision deteriorated from 6/9 to 1/60, although it improved later and stabilized at 6/18. (a) An upper temporal branch vein occlusion with vascular sheathing. (b) Large areas of nonperfusion are demonstrated over the upper temporal quadrant and the affected vein and its branches are irregular. One branch is slow to fill and is seen as a hypofluorescent masking line. (c) In the late picture, the vessel walls show intense hyperfluorescence with fuzzy outlines where they pass through areas of capillary closure. The risk of neovascularization between 1–3 years after the occlusion is high in such a case, and this patient was eventually treated with sectoral scatter retinal photocoagulation when disc new vessels developed.

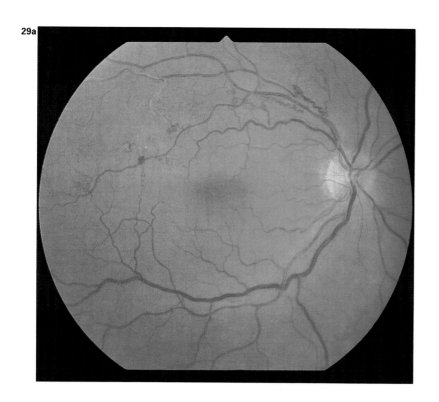

Indications for angiography

Angiography is rarely required for diagnosis in acute cases but is used, as in branch vein occlusion, to determine the precise cause of the visual loss, and the extent of retinal nonperfusion.

Determination of cause of visual loss Vascular abnormalities in the macular area are almost always present in the acute stage. Spontaneous improvement does occur, particularly in the younger age group, but permanent loss of central vision usually occurs as a result of foveal ischaemia, retinal pigment epithelial atrophy or persistent oedema (**31**).

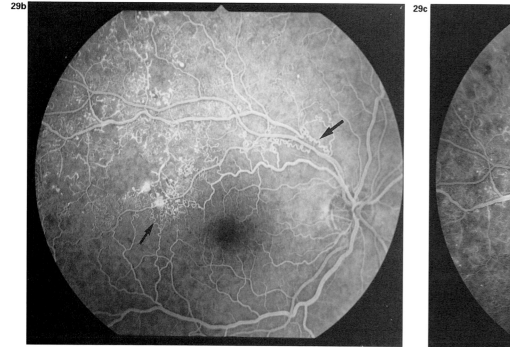

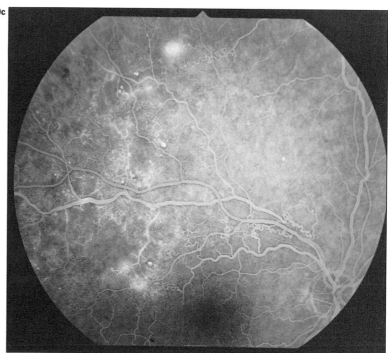

29 Branch retinal vein occlusion: collateral vessels. This woman had presented at the age of 48 with a right retinal branch vein occlusion. She had been found to have a blood pressure of 250/150 and was admitted for emergency treatment. She later suffered a branch vein occlusion in her other eye. The angiogram was performed 11 years after the acute episode. (**a**) In this long-standing vein occlusion, tortuous collateral vessels have developed. (**b,c**) Angiography confirms the presence of many collateral channels (arrows). Unlike disc or retinal new vessels, collaterals do not leak dye. However, the distinction is usually easy to make on ophthalmoscopy, and angiography is rarely necessary under these circumstances.

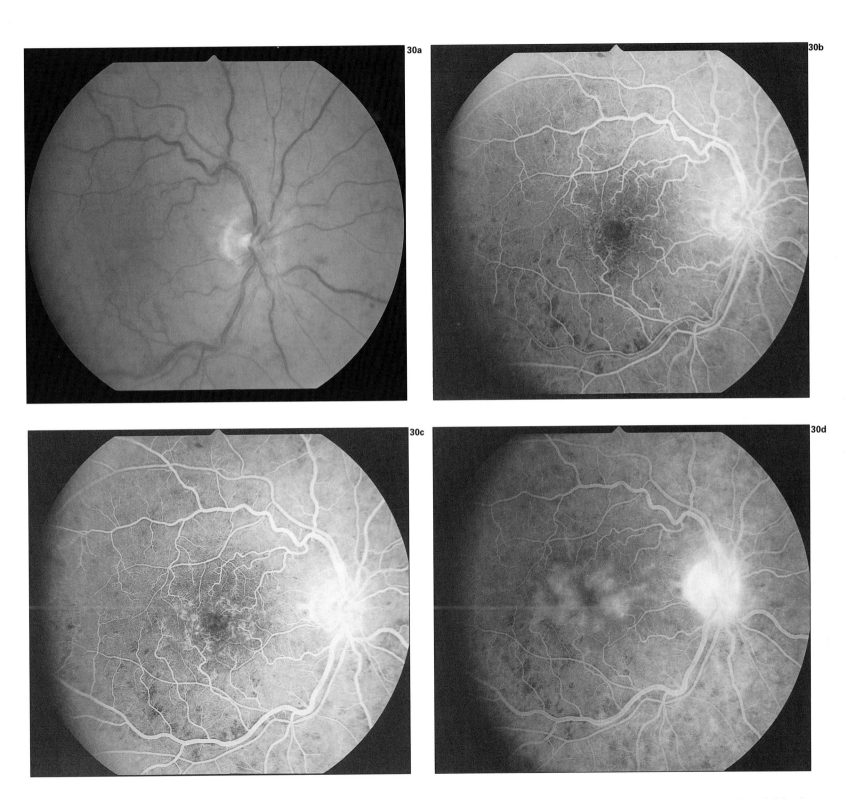

30 Central retinal vein occlusion: hyperpermeability. A 66-year-old woman with a history of hypertension and ischaemic heart disease noticed blurring of vision in her left eye and a visual acuity of 6/18 was recorded. Over the next few months it improved to 6/9. (**a**) Central retinal vein occlusion. (**b,c,d**) The macular capillary bed appears well perfused but dilated and permeable. The risk of neovascular complications is very small, but vision is reduced by exudation. There is leakage from the capillaries adjacent to the capillary-free zone, and the late picture (**d**) shows the characteristic pattern of cystoid macular oedema. The intense late fluorescence of the disc and its indistinct borders indicate leakage.

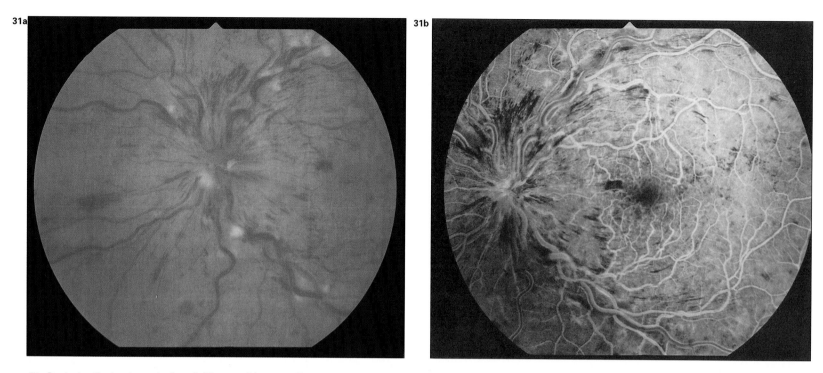

31 Central retinal vein occlusion. A 61-year-old man suffered a rapid deterioration of vision in his left eye. His visual acuity at the time of the angiogram was 6/60 and over the following year improved to 6/24. (**a**) This case shows a more florid picture with tortuous vessels and cotton wool spots. (**b**) The capillary bed in this area of fundus is well perfused.

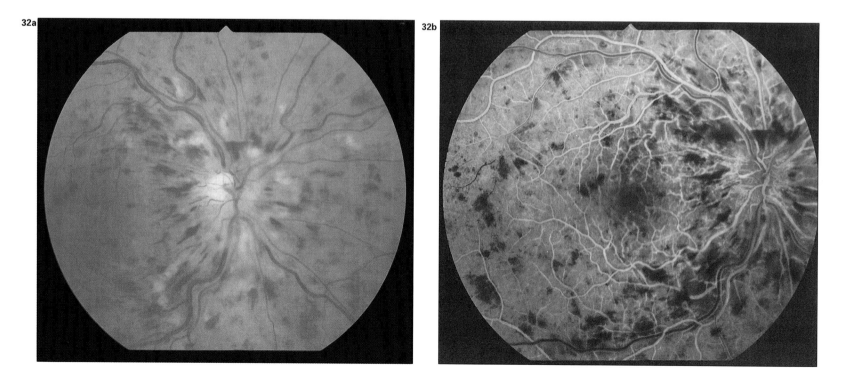

Assessment of extent of nonperfusion Approximately two-thirds of cases of central retinal vein occlusion show diffuse hyperpermeability and one-third show some degree of retinal ischaemia (**32,33**—also **24**). Early detection of widespread nonperfusion is of particular importance in central retinal vein occlusion because of the serious consequences of the development of neovascular glaucoma. The presence of large diffuse haemorrhages, many cotton wool spots and a profound loss of vision, is suggestive of widespread retinal nonperfusion, although clinical appearance alone is not a reliable indicator, and absence of any of these features does not rule out significant ischaemia. The area of retinal capillary filling defects demonstrated by angiography has important prognostic significance—it has been shown that an area of nonperfusion approximately 50% or more of a 30° fundus photograph leads to neovascular glaucoma in 40–60% of cases.

Panretinal photocoagulation has been shown to prevent iris neovascularisation, or promote regression of existing new vessels. As neovascular glaucoma can occur within weeks of the original occlusion, fluorescein angiography should be performed within 4–6 weeks of the onset of symptoms. Assessment of the capillary bed can be difficult where extensive haemorrhage persists, but usually there are areas which are not obscured and can be evaluated. However, very early angiography (within a few days of onset of symptoms) is often unhelpful, particularly in the presence of vitreous haemorrhage or widespread retinal haemorrhage, and may be misleading in those cases where the pattern of ischaemia is still evolving.

The information from an angiogram is used to assess the risk of neovascularization (see p. 21). If the risk is high, prophylactic panretinal photocoagulation is considered, or frequent follow-up visits arranged.

Retinal arterial occlusions

Angiograms are not necessary for the diagnosis of branch or central retinal arterial occlusions (**34,35**). In the acute phase the symptoms of sudden visual loss, pallor of the infarcted retina, a broken stream of blood within the affected vessels (*cattle-trucking*) and occasionally visible emboli, present an easily recognisable clinical picture. Once these signs are no longer present, and if there is no obvious arterial narrowing or sheathing, an angiogram provides little if any additional information. Filling of the retinal vessels often returns to normal after an acute event, particularly if an embolus moves along the circulation.

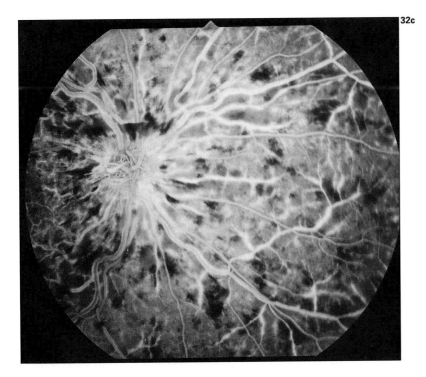

32c

32 Central retinal vein occlusion: moderate nonperfusion. A fit man of 66 noticed sudden loss of vision in his right eye. His visual acuity at presentation was 1/60 and there was a right afferent pupillary defect. (**a**) A similar appearance to **31**. (**b**) In this case, there is perfusion of the capillary bed at the macula, but there are large areas of featureless nonperfused retina temporally. (**c**) Interpretation of the vascular pattern is more difficult in these later pictures of the nasal retina. Many of the smaller order vessels are patent but there are definite small patches of capillary nonperfusion, and other areas where it is suspected. Vessel walls exhibit intense hyperfluorescence where they pass through ischaemic retina.

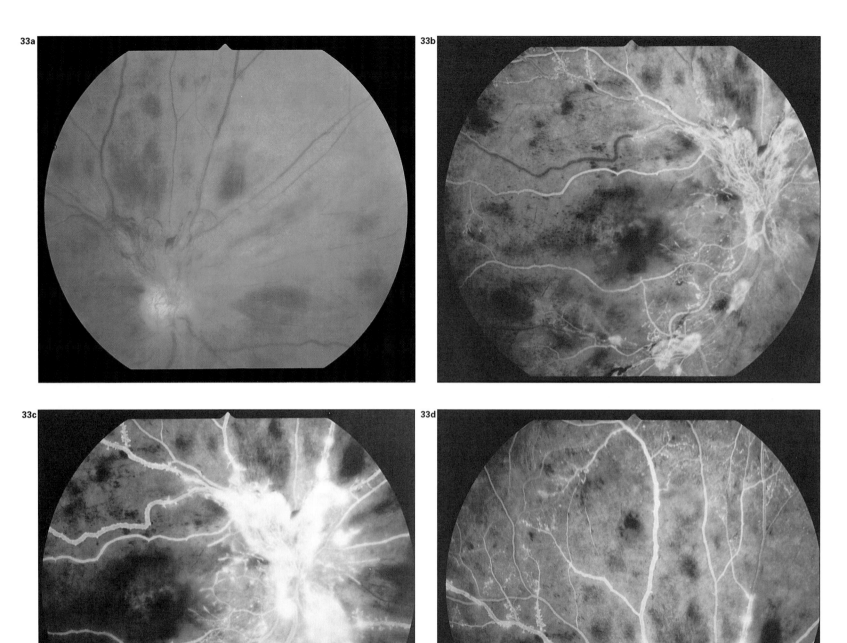

33 Central retinal vein occlusion: ischaemia, neovascularization. A 65-year-old man noticed profound loss of vision in his right eye. (**a**) Three months following onset of symptoms, fundus neovascularization was observed. (**b,c,d**) There is no filling of retinal capillaries over most of the area photographed. There is a network of new disc and retinal vessels which leak with intense fluorescence in the late pictures. An interesting feature is the budding of tiny vessels from the walls of the branches of the superior temporal branch vein, early signs of intraretinal neovascularization. (See also **24**.)

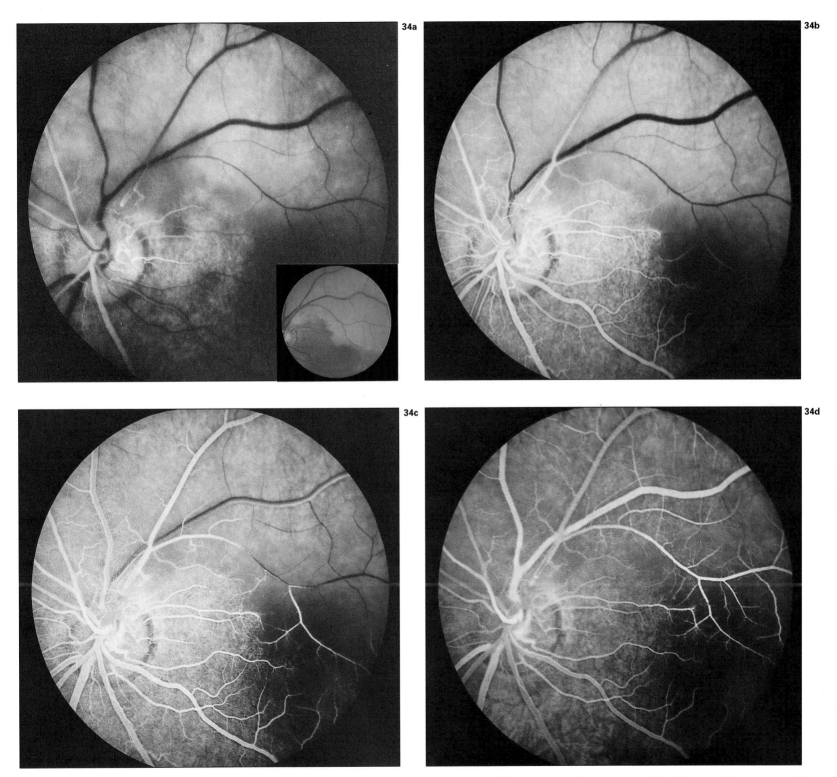

34 Branch retinal artery occlusion. A young woman aged 18 presented with sudden loss of vision. She was otherwise asymptomatic. A late systolic murmur and bigeminy of the pulse was demonstrated and an embolus arising from the heart was suspected as a cause for her visual symptoms. **(Inset)** Occlusion of the upper temporal arteriole. **(a,b,c,d)** The contrast between perfused and nonperfused retina is demonstrated. There are cilioretinal vessels which fill early, and there is evidence of retrograde flow from the area they supply into the arteriolar branches of the occluded branch artery. Note the origin of the superior temporal arteriole which does not fill with dye but which appears normal on the colour photograph.

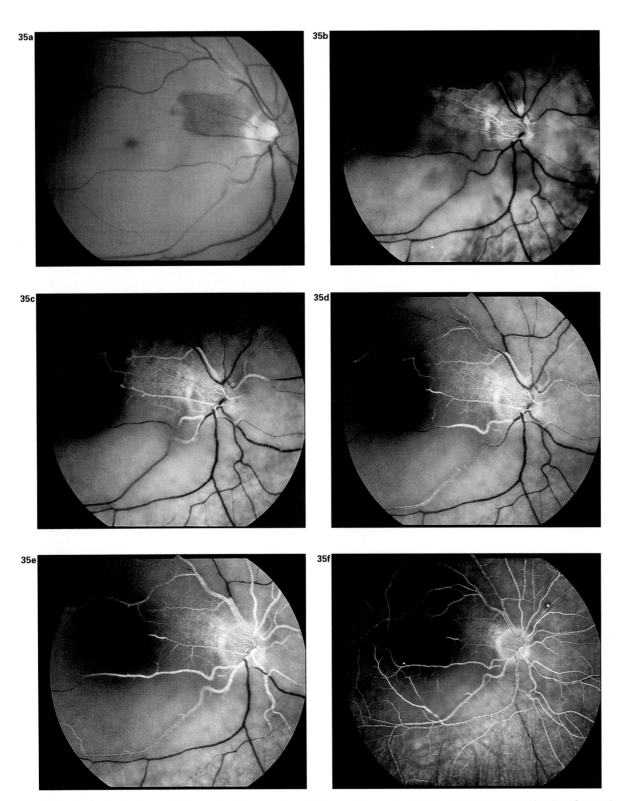

35 Central retinal artery occlusion with ciliary sparing. A 38-year-old man presented with sudden loss of vision. Systemic investigation revealed a prolapsing mitral valve. (**a**) Central retinal artery occlusion with ciliary sparing. (**b**) Normal choroidal fluorescence is present and a patent cilioretinal artery fills at the same time as the choroid. The capillaries on the surface of the disc fill from the choroidal supply to the circle of Zinn. Fluorescence of a branch of the superior temporal vein draining the perfused area is noted before any dye appears in the retinal arteries. (**c**) 20 seconds. (**d**) 38 seconds. (**e**) 60 seconds. (**f**) Two minutes. Retrograde filling of a retinal arteriole is seen in (c) and (d). (c–f) show the very slow fill of the retinal vessels. Normal retinal capillary hyperfluorescence is seen only in the territory of the cilioretinal artery. The choroidal vascular pattern is more distinct in contrast to the area just below and temporal to the disc where there is masking by the opacified, infarcted retina.

Retinopathy in systemic disease

Diabetic retinopathy

Fluorescein angiography initially played an important role in the development of the understanding of the vascular changes in diabetic retinopathy (**36–43**). As a result a rationale for treatment was developed, providing guidelines for the planning and monitoring of photocoagulation therapy. As the appearances of diabetic retinopathy and their angiographic correlates have become more familiar, many practitioners now feel confident enough to treat without a preliminary angiogram, reserving the investigation for cases where additional information is required, particularly in the treatment of maculopathy.

Indications for angiography

Determination of cause of visual loss It is sometimes difficult to explain the cause of visual deterioration in a diabetic patient, particularly in the elderly. Fluorescein angiography enables differentiation between macular nonperfusion (**39**) and macular oedema due to hyperpermeability of the retinal capillaries (**37,40**), and reveals the presence of additional, unrelated pathology (e.g. subretinal neovascularization). Angiography is particularly useful in cases which do not seem to follow an expected clinical course either before or after laser treatment.

Assessment of degree of retinal ischaemia There are many clinical features which point to the presence of significant ischaemia, such as venous beading or loops, diffuse haemorrhages, sheathed vessels, numerous cotton wool spots, intraretinal microvascular abnormalities (IRMA) and retinal and disc neovascularization (**41,42,43**). The presence of disc new vessels or forward-growing retinal new vessels implies widespread retinal nonperfusion and is an indication for photocoagulation without the need for fluorescein angiography. In preproliferative retinopathy, an assessment of the extent of inner retinal nonperfusion is believed to be useful in predicting the likelihood of neovascularisation, and some clinicians advocate early treatment in those patients at high risk.

Treatment of maculopathy There are two main causes of visual deterioration in diabetic maculopathy—ischaemia and hyperpermeability.

If the cause of visual loss is impaired perfusion (**39**), photocoagulation is not beneficial.

Hyperpermeability may be focal or diffuse. Focal leakage produces patches of retinal thickening associated with vascular abnormalities. There are often exudates, which develop in rings or part-rings with the microvascular anomaly in the centre. The source of leakage is determined on biomicroscopy. There is little evidence that angiography in such cases improves the result of photocoagulation therapy.

Angiography is useful in cases of diffuse hyperpermeability to exclude foveal ischaemia and determine areas of more pronounced leakage. Grid photocoagulation has a role if foveal ischaemia is not present.

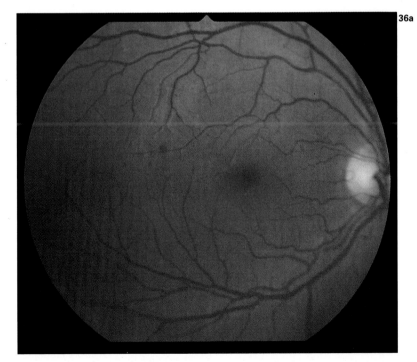
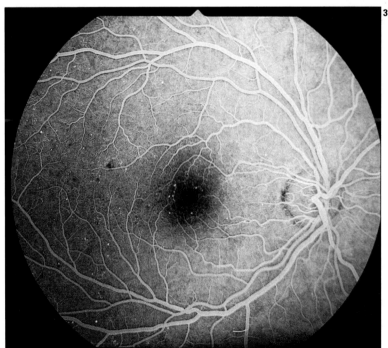

36 Diabetic retinopathy (mild background) in a 45-year-old insulin-dependent diabetic. The patient was asymptomatic, with a visual acuity of 6/5. (**a**) Mild background retinopathy with microaneurysms and small haemorrhages. (**b**) Microaneurysms appear as fluorescent dots and the haemorrhages as small patches of masking. Minimal disturbance of the capillary bed is demonstrated.

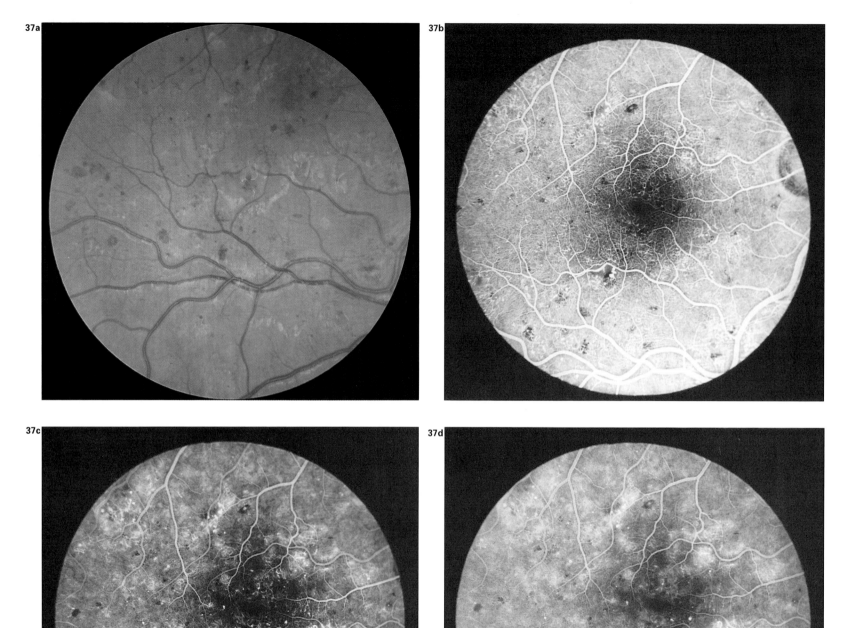

37 Diabetic retinopathy – background. This woman had been an insulin-dependent diabetic for eight years. Visual acuity was 6/6, 6/5. (**a**) Fundoscopy showed microaneurysms, scattered small haemorrhages and one cotton wool spot (**b**). Patches of hypofluorescence correspond with haemorrhages. There is widening of intercapillary spaces at the macula and areas of capillary dilatation can be seen, particularly around small patches of non-perfusion. (**c,d**) Patches of leakage from the affected capillaries and some microaneurysms.

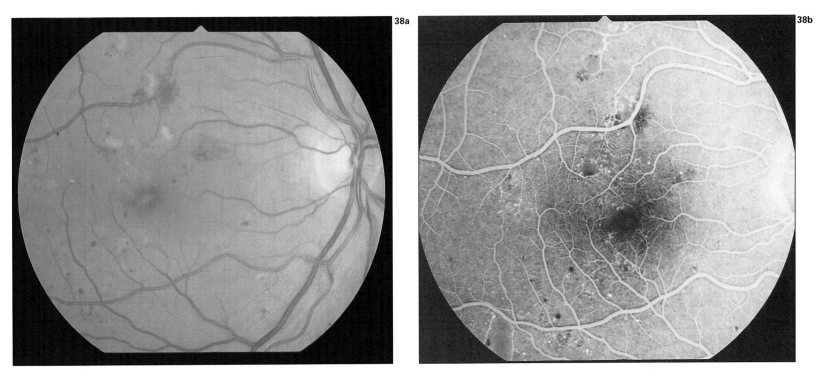

38 Diabetic retinopathy – background. (**a**) In addition to haemorrhages, microaneurysms and fine exudates, there are several cotton wool spots. (**b**) Small capillary filling defects correspond in position with the cotton wool spots demonstrated in (**a**).

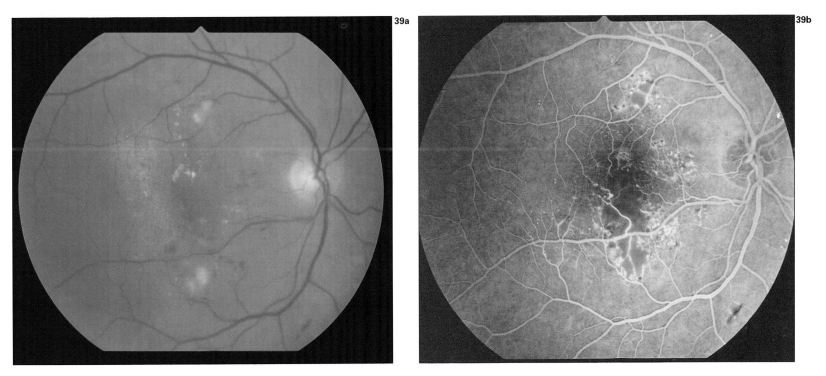

39 Diabetic retinopathy – ischaemic maculopathy. A 65-year-old man with non-insulin-dependent diabetes presented with VA 6/18 in the right eye. (**a**) Cotton wool spots and scattered exudates are present. (**b**) There is an area of nonperfusion immediately below the central fovea which doubtless contributes significantly to the reduction in vision.

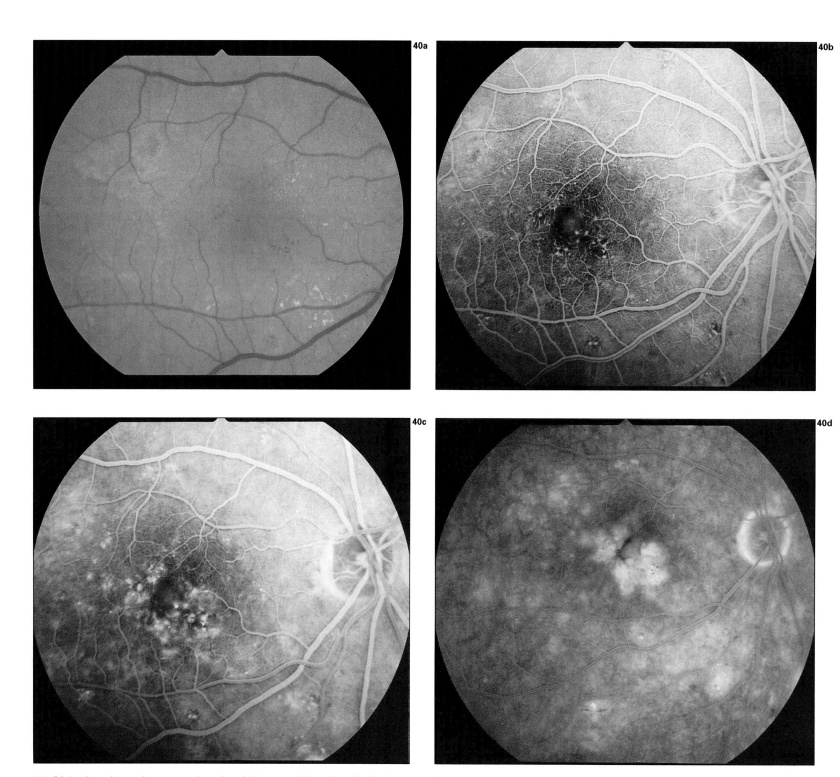

40 Diabetic retinopathy – maculopathy. A 74-year-old non-insulin-dependent diabetic suffered a drop in visual acuity in the right eye to 6/12. (**a**) There are haemorrhages, exudates and microaneurysms. The difficulty of demonstrating macular oedema on colour photographs is emphasized. (**b,c**) There is leakage from the perifoveal capillary bed. (**d**) In the late pictures, the characteristic petaloid pattern of cystoid macular oedema appears.

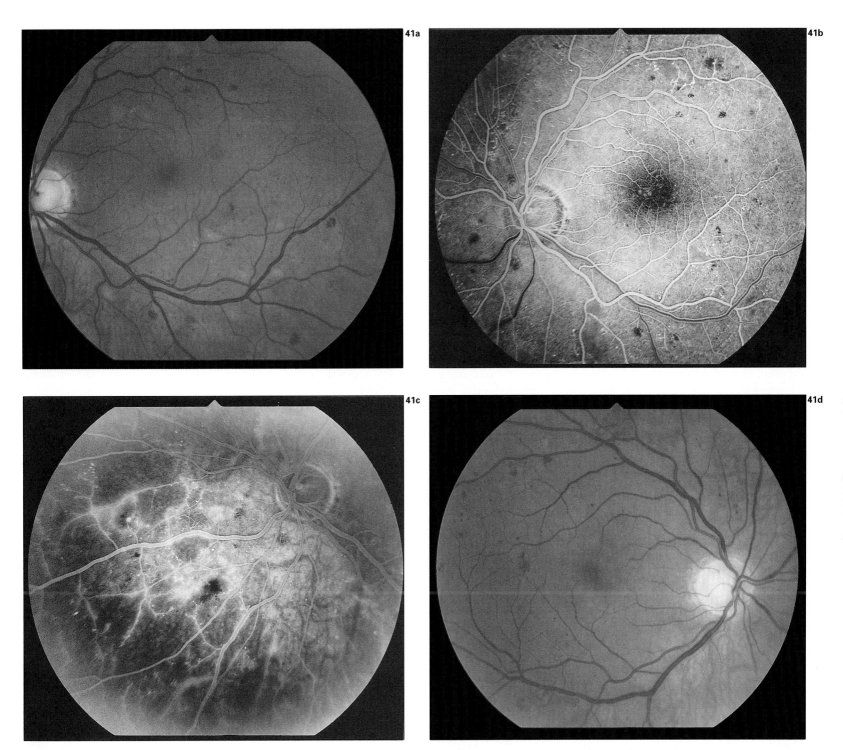

41 Diabetic retinopathy – preproliferative. This 37-year-old diabetic had noticed a deterioration in his left vision (VA 6/6, 6/12). (**a**) Cotton wool spots and blotchy haemorrhages in the left eye. (**b**) The macula is well perfused. There are small filling defects surrounded by budding capillaries beside the temporal vessels. (**c**) The nonperfusion of the capillary bed is much more widespread in the peripheral retina. (**d**) The other eye already shows retinal neovascularization.

42a

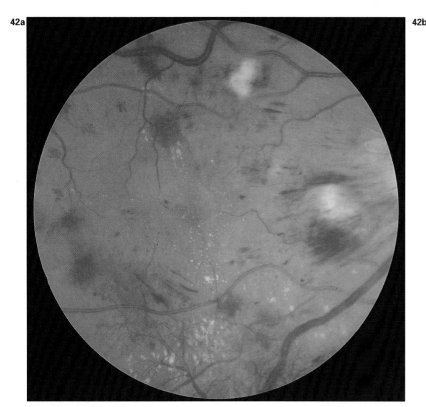

42b

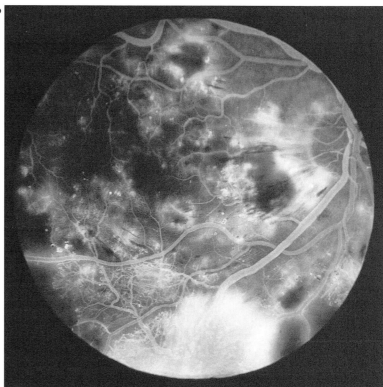

42c

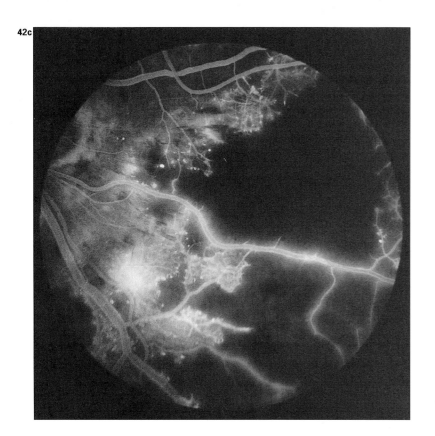

42 Diabetic retinopathy – proliferative. A 52-year-old man had been treated for diabetes for 11 years. He presented with blurred vision in the left eye, VA 6/5, CF. (**a**) The left eye showed dense vitreous haemorrhage. On the right there was advanced retinopathy with neovascularization. (**b**) Florid retinal neovascularization. (**c**) Extensive filling defects of the nasal retinal vasculature.

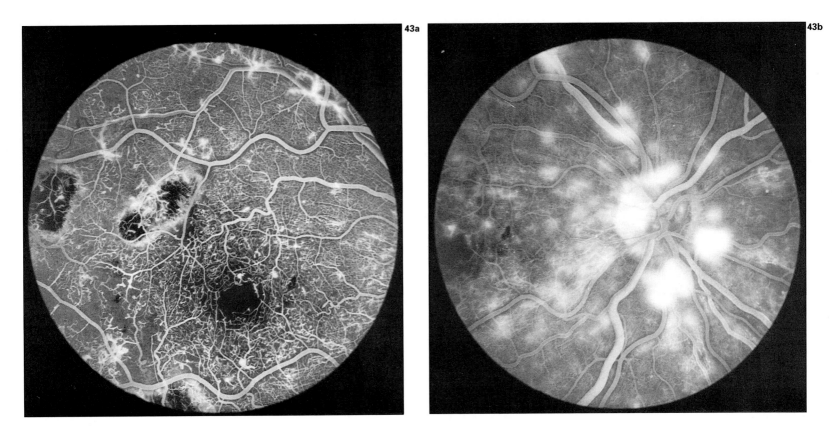

43 Diabetic retinopathy – proliferative. A 35-year-old insulin-dependent diabetic who also suffered from nephropathy had undergone panretinal photocoagulation, but neovascularization persisted. **(a)** The macular capillary bed is abnormal with widening of the intercapillary spaces and irregularity of the margins of the foveal avascular zone. There are areas of capillary closure with budding of the surrounding capillaries and preretinal new vessels. Two areas of hypofluorescence mark the position of photocoagulation scars. **(b)** Late pictures show leakage from disc and retinal new vessels, causing intense hyperfluorescence.

Hypertension

Uncontrolled systemic hypertension affects both the retinal and choroidal vasculature (**44,45**). The first change in response to an elevation in blood pressure is retinal arteriolar constriction. In prolonged hypertension the walls of the arterioles thicken, with narrowing of the lumen and an increase in their external calibre. At the arteriovenous crossings, where the arteriole and venule share a common adventitial sheath, compression of the venule occurs to give the sign known as 'nipping'. At this stage angiography shows a normal capillary bed with no evidence of breakdown of the blood–retinal barrier.

In more severe cases the microvasculature is affected, with the development of microaneurysms, cotton wool spots, haemorrhages and exudates. In accelerated or malignant hypertension, swelling of the optic disc occurs (**44**). Involvement of choroidal arterioles leads to patchy nonperfusion of the choroid (**45**) and ischaemia of the overlying pigment epithelium. The outer blood–retinal barrier breaks down, sometimes resulting in localized retinal detachments.

Other conditions closely associated with hypertension are branch vein occlusion, retinal macroaneurysms and ischaemic optic neuritis. A too rapid reduction of the blood pressure, particularly in children, can also be associated with optic nerve ischaemia.

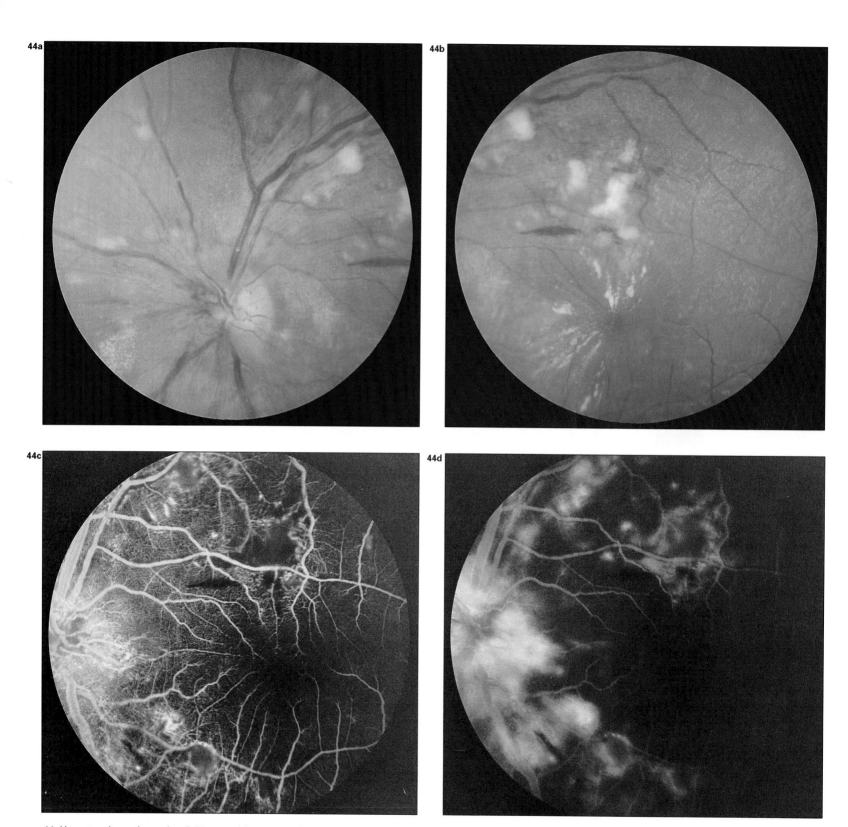

44 Hypertensive retinopathy. A 25-year-old man complained of blurred vision which was recorded as 6/12 in each eye. His blood pressure was 270/180. (**a,b**) He was found to have bilateral disc swelling, cotton wool spots and haemorrhages, and a macular star in his left eye. (**c,d**) The larger vessels are irregular in calibre. There are patches of capillary dilatation and closure. There is leakage of dye from the disc and from areas of abnormal retinal vasculature.

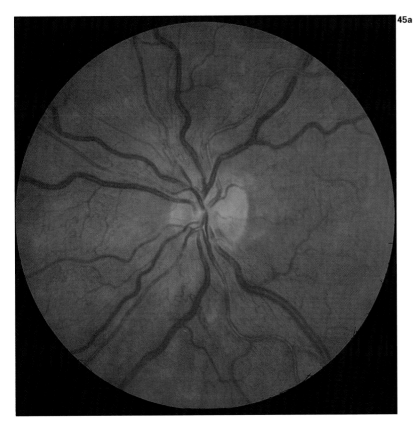

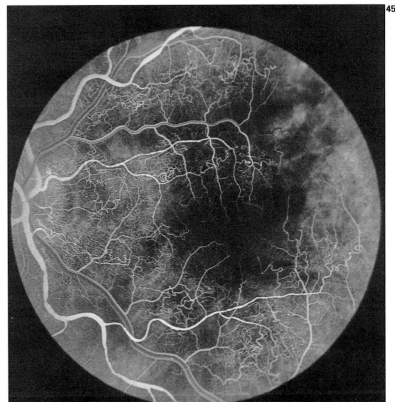

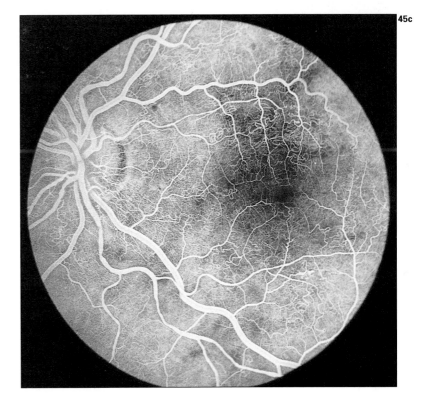

45 Hypertensive retinopathy. A 42-year-old man noticed visual disturbance and headache. His blood pressure was 260/180 and there was albumin in his urine. (**a**) The retinal veins are dilated, and the arterioles appear narrow with a heightened central reflex. Arteriovenous nipping is demonstrated. There are no microaneurysms, haemorrhages, exudates or oedema and the disc is not swollen. (**b,c**) There is marked constriction of the retinal arterioles and tortuosity of the smaller order arterioles and capillaries. Patchy background hypofluorescence suggests the presence of choroidal filling defects. There is no leakage of dye from the retinal vessels or the disc.

Sickle cell retinopathy

Sickle cell haemoglobinopathies are characterized by the production of an abnormal haemoglobin which affects the normal function of erythrocytes. Under conditions of reduced oxygenation, the cells become sickle shaped and rigid and are unable to pass through smaller vessels. The abnormality has been traced to a defective gene which leads to production of haemoglobin S in the place of normal adult haemoglobin A. Homozygous sickle cell disease (SS) is associated with serious systemic manifestations caused by vascular occlusion, haemolysis and infection. In the heterozygous condition, the gene for haemoglobin S is inherited from one parent, and a gene for haemoglobin C, thalassaemia or normal haemoglobin A from the other. In SC and S-thal disease the systemic manifestations are milder than in SS disease, but ocular complications are more pronounced. In AS disease, or sickle-cell trait, both ocular and systemic manifestations are rare.

Ocular manifestations

Various ocular structures including the conjunctiva, the iris and the optic disc may be involved in sickle cell disease, but it is the retina that is primarily affected (**46**).

Sickle cell retinopathy Occlusion of peripheral retinal arterioles leads to ischaemia of the peripheral retina. Severity of retinopathy ranges from mild signs of vascular occlusion, to proliferative changes, haemorrhages and detachments. Five stages of retinopathy are described:

I   Peripheral arteriolar occlusion.
II Peripheral arteriovenous anastomosis.
III Peripheral retinal neovascularisation (sea-fan configuration).
IV Vitreous haemorrhage.
V   Retinal detachment.

Although the retinopathy characteristically affects the periphery, the posterior pole is sometimes involved. There may be tortuosity of the large vessels and occlusion of macular arterioles.

The salmon patch lesion is a haemorrhage of an orange-yellow colour within the sensory retina, which develops after sudden occlusion of a medium-sized arteriole. It resolves leaving a retinoschisis cavity. The chorioretinal scars known as black sunbursts are thought to develop from salmon patches.

Epiretinal membranes occur in about 4% of cases of sickle cell retinopathy and are an important cause of maculopathy. They are more frequent following treatment of proliferative changes with photocoagulation, which in certain cases may be a factor in their causation.

Angioid streaks are common but appear to carry a more benign prognosis than those seen in pseudoxanthoma elasticum. Macular neovascularization is rare.

Uses of angiography

Fluorescein angiography is useful in determining the extent of peripheral vascular closure when planning photocoagulation treatment in proliferative sickle cell retinopathy. Prophylactic treatment has not been found to be effective, but scatter photocoagulation around a sea fan leads to the regression of small lesions. It is suggested, though not yet proven, that photocoagulation scattered over wider areas of ischaemic retina may prove even more effective.

Angiography is useful in determining the cause of central visual loss which is not obviously related to the severity of peripheral changes. It can detect macular nonperfusion, and the vascular distortion caused by shrinkage of epiretinal membranes. It is essential if neovascular membranes associated with angioid streaks are to be treated.

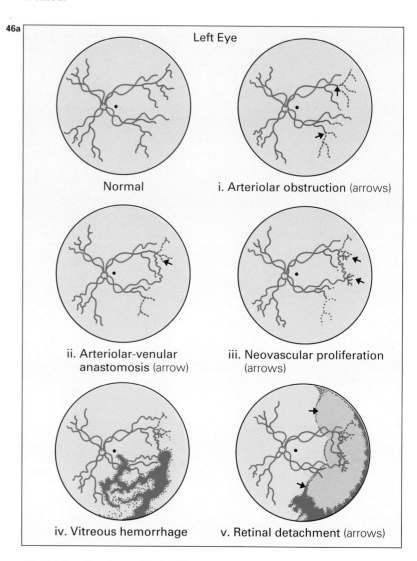

46a

46 Sickle cell retinopathy. (**a**) Diagram illustrating the stages of sickle cell retinopathy. (**b**) Stage 1 sickle cell retinopathy: colour photograph and fluorescein angiogram demonstrating peripheral arterial closure. (**c**) A large peripheral neovascular lesion with the characteristic sea fan configuration. (**d**) Angiogram demonstrating sea fans and arteriovenous communications. The neovascular lesions leak profusely in the late stages of the angiogram. (**e**) Angiograms one year apart demonstrating autoinfarction of a large sea fan lesion. (**f**) Angiograms showing disappearance of a large sea fan lesion following gentle scatter coagulation. (**g**) Proliferative sickle cell retinopathy with early vitreoretinal traction. The patient developed a retinal detachment but unfortunately the visual acuity did not improve following surgery. (Courtesy of Mr P I Condon, Waterford, Ireland, and Professor G Serjeant, Kingston, Jamaica.)

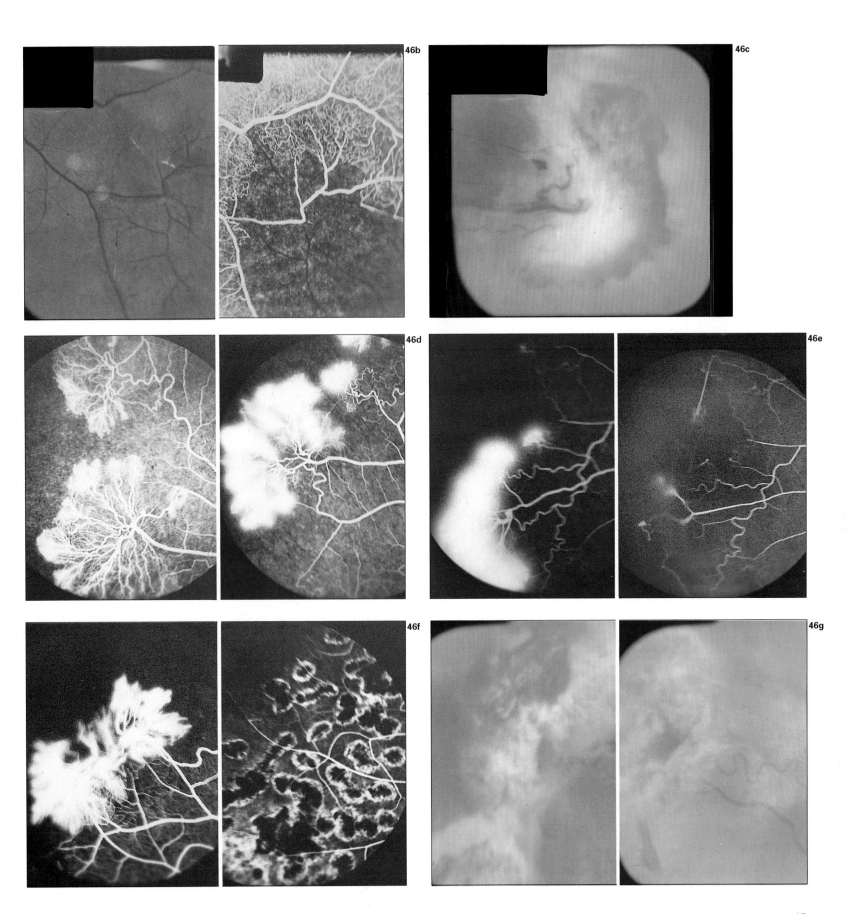

45

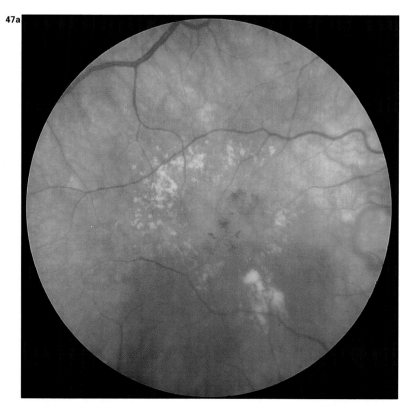

Other retinal vascular disorders

Radiation retinopathy

Although the neuroretina is resistant to radiation damage, the retinal vasculature is susceptible and radiation retinopathy is a well-recognized complication of radiotherapy to the eye, orbit and surrounding structures (**47**).

The progression of radiation retinopathy is typically very slow. Damage to endothelial cells initially leads to the formation of microaneurysms, capillary irregularities and small areas of nonperfusion. Larger areas of nonperfusion develop with associated areas of telangiectasia. Hyperpermeability of the abnormal vasculature results in retinal oedema and widespread inner retinal nonperfusion to retinal, preretinal and disc neovascularization. Choroidal infarction and ischaemic optic neuropathy are also reported. The severity of radiation retinopathy appears to be more pronounced in cases with pre-existing microangiopathy, for example diabetic retinopathy and concomitant chemotherapy. Angiography is used to assess the severity of radiation damage, to determine the cause of visual loss and to estimate the extent and location of areas of nonperfusion.

Retinal macroaneurysms

Retinal macroaneurysms are not uncommon in the elderly population, particularly in women. They are usually unilateral and solitary, affect-

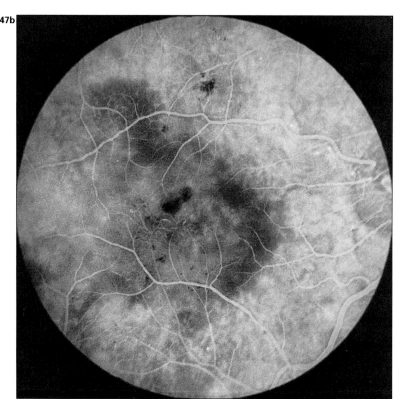

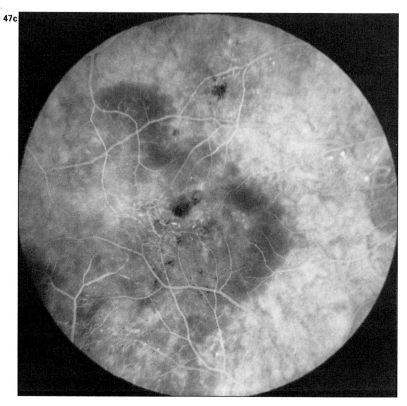

47 Radiation retinopathy. A 17-year-old man had undergone radiotherapy and chemotherapy three years previously for carcinoma of the nasopharynx. He became aware of a right central scotoma (VA 6/24, 6/6). (**a**) Oedema and haemorrhage at the macula with a surrounding ring of exudate. (**b,c**) There is coarsening of the capillary network at the macula with leakage of dye. Reduction in background fluorescence which persists through the transit suggests choroidal involvement.

ing second- or third-order arterioles, but may be multiple or bilateral. There is often no evidence of other ocular disease, but a strong association exists with hypertension and/or generalized cardiovascular disease. Visual loss arises when exudation or haemorrhage affects the foveal area, or if vitreous haemorrhage occurs. Partial rupture of the aneurysm produces a leak at arteriolar pressure at a retinal, subretinal or preretinal level which is often extensive. Macroaneurysms should be considered as a cause in all cases of vitreous haemorrhage in elderly patients. Treatment with photocoagulation is reserved for those cases where central vision is threatened by oedema or exudate.

A macroaneurysm appears on ophthalmoscopy as a round dilatation over or beside a retinal arteriole. Colour ranges from red to pale yellow. On angiography, the aneurysm fills with dye at the same time as the adjacent retinal arteriole. In late pictures, staining of the wall and leakage from the aneurysm leads to persisting hyperfluorescence (48). Capillary dilatation and non-perfusion are frequently seen around the lesion, and there may be closure of the arteriole beyond.

Angiography is particularly helpful where there is doubt about the diagnosis, for example in the presence of extensive haemorrhage. A macroaneurysm may be mistaken for a branch vein occlusion, for instance, and indeed the two conditions are sometimes found in association. Under these circumstances, angiography delineates the characteristic shape of the aneurysm as it fills with dye, distinguishing it from surrounding haemorrhage and oedema. However, fluorescein angiography is often of limited use in cases which cause most problems in diagnosis, because of the masking effect of the haemorrhage.

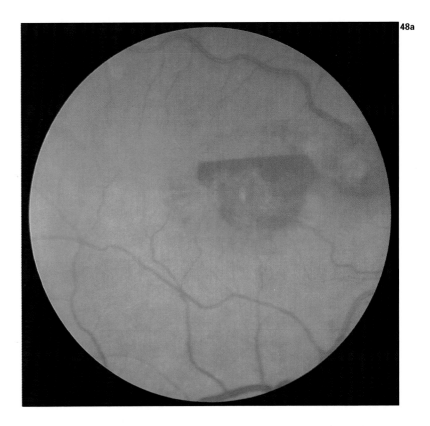

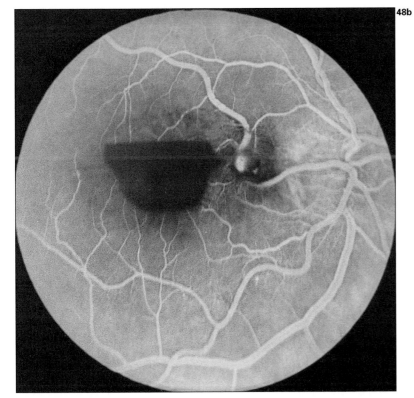

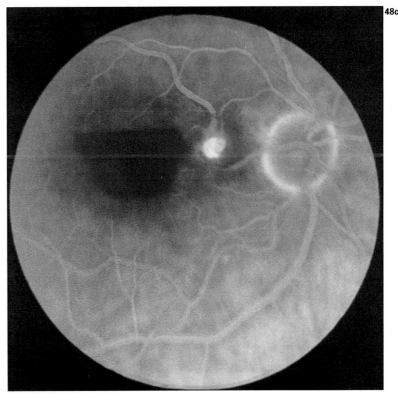

48 Retinal macroaneurysm. A 75-year-old woman who was being treated for hypertension noticed a sudden reduction in her central vision. (a) A preretinal haemorrhage at the macula. The macroaneurysm is difficult to distinguish from the surrounding retinal haemorrhage. (b) The macroaneurysm is clearly demonstrated on angiography. (c) The lesion remains hyperfluorescent in the late frames due to leakage of dye and staining of its walls.

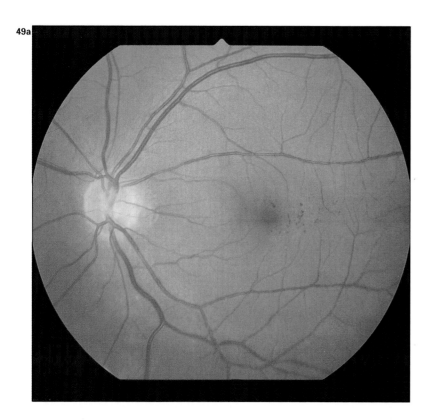

Parafoveal telangiectasia

This condition is congenital or acquired (**49**). Similar appearances may be secondary to venous occlusion or radiation retinopathy. In other cases, it may represent part of the spectrum of disorders which include Coats' disease. Visual loss occurs when oedema or exudate involve the central fovea, and fluorescein angiography is useful to identify the extent of the telangiectatic vessels if treatment with photocoagulation is to be contemplated.

Coats' disease

Fluorescein angiography has played an important part in the understanding of the vascular morphology of Coats' disease, and is useful in planning and monitoring treatment by photocoagulation. The massive retinal exudation characteristic of the disorder arises from areas of telangiectasia and aneurysmal dilatation of larger retinal vessels (**50**). Photocoagulation of these vessels where appropriate leads to resolution of the exudates and subretinal fluid.

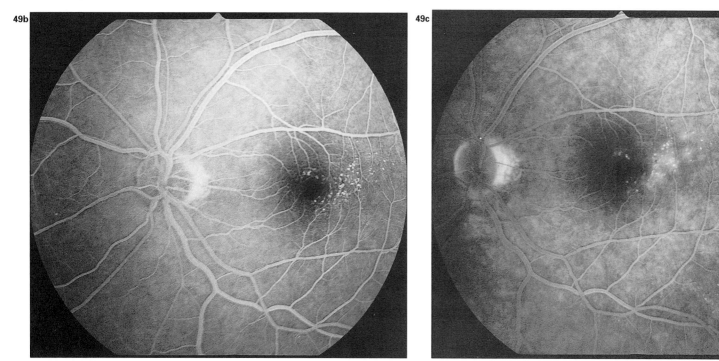

49 Parafoveal telangiectasia. A 49-year-old man was asymptomatic with a visual acuity of 6/6, but his optician noted abnormal vessels at his left macula. (**a,b**) Telangiectasia of the capillary bed temporal to the foveola. (**c**) The late picture shows leakage of the affected vessels.

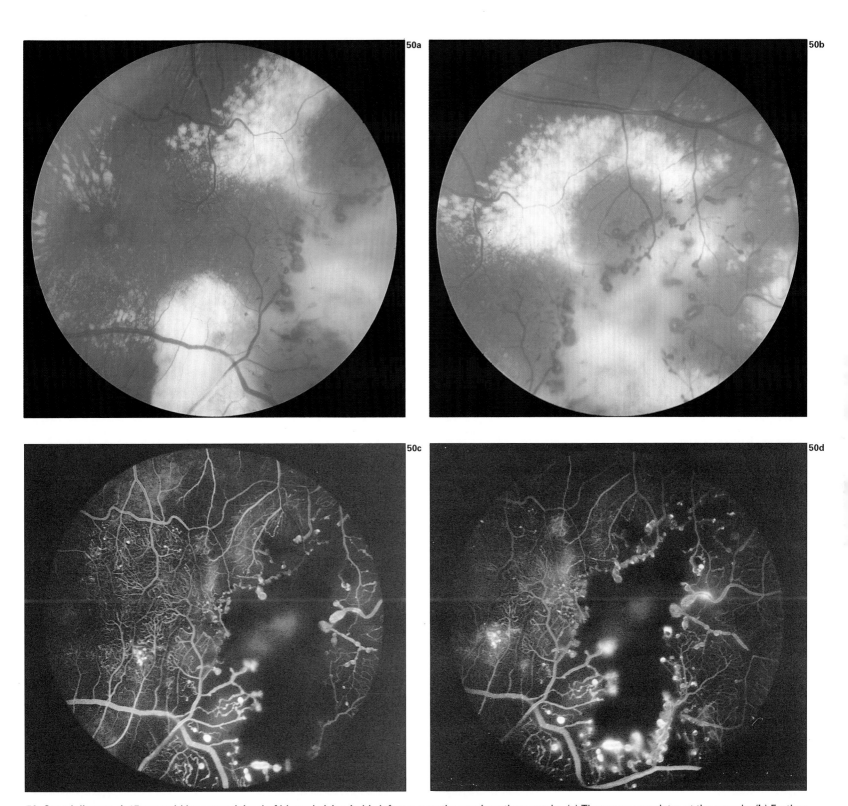

50 Coats' disease. A 15-year-old boy complained of blurred vision in his left eye over the previous three weeks. **(a)** There were exudates at the macula. **(b)** Further exudates in the temporal periphery were associated with telangiectasia. **(c)** A patch of capillary nonperfusion surrounded by abnormal vessels which show vascular beading, dilatations and abnormal communications. The capillary bed to the left of the ischaemic area shows coarsening of the network and scattered microaneurysms. This frame corresponds with the view in **(b)**. **(d)** There is leakage of dye from many of the abnormal dilatations.

Racemose haemangioma

Retinal vascular malformations with abnormal arteriovenous communications are known as racemose haemangiomas. They occur in isolation or as part of the Wyburn–Mason syndrome, where they may be associated with intracranial aneurysms. The lesion can be small and confined to a small area of the fundus, but in more severe cases it is spectacular with marked dilatation and tortuosity of the retinal vessels (**51**). Even on angiography, it may be difficult to distinguish venous from arterial channels.

Retinal capillary haemangioma (von Hippel tumour)

Fluorescein angiography is helpful in differentiating a peripheral angioma from other causes of exudation (e.g. retinal macroaneurysm, Coats' disease or diabetic retinopathy) and other causes of peripheral arteriovenous communications. It is important to identify the lesions at an early stage, as treatment with photocoagulation or cryotherapy may prevent sight-threatening complications. Retinal haemangiomas are also often the earliest manifestation of the dominantly inherited von Hippel–Lindau disease and alert the clinician to the possibility of associated neurological and renal lesions.

The tumour is single or multiple. It is composed of a mass of large-diameter capillaries which act as shunts and lead to enlargement of the afferent and efferent vessels (**52**). As the lesion develops, the capillaries become permeable, and exudation occurs. Overlying fibrovascular proliferation and traction eventually lead to vitreous haemorrhage and retinal detachment.

Screening for von Hippel lesions in those patients with a family history is usually performed using ophthalmoscopy. Fluorescein angiography is used to confirm the diagnosis where it is in doubt.

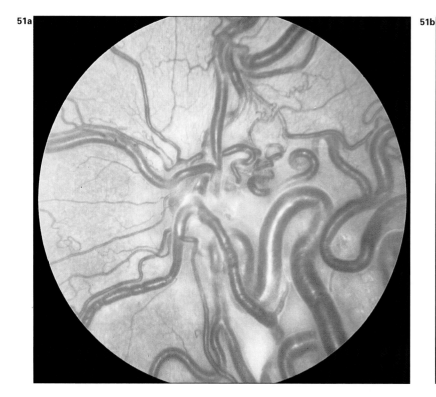
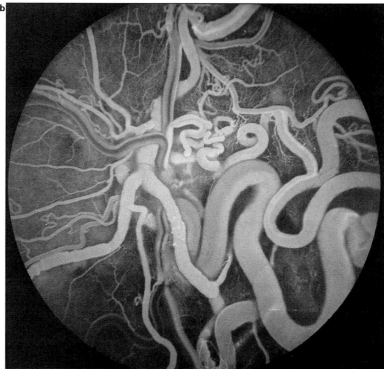

51 Congenital arteriovenous communication, racemose haemangioma. (**a,b**) Surprisingly, visual acuity was 6/24 in this case. The other eye was normal.

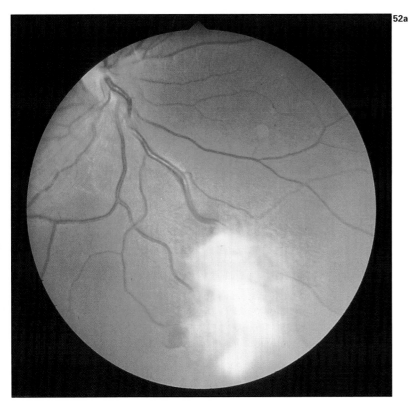
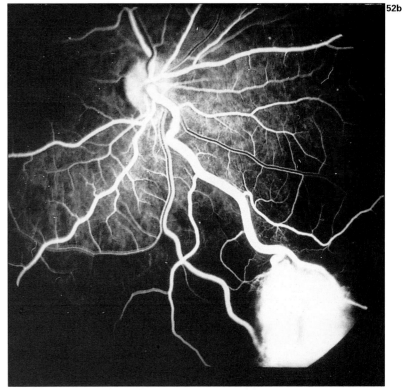

52 Peripheral retinal capillary haemangioma (von Hippel tumour). (**a,b**) Enlargement of the feeder and draining vessel is demonstrated. The lesion is intensely hyperfluorescent at this early stage of the transit with leakage of dye. Details of the capillary structure of the tumour are obscured. (Courtesy of Miss Carol Lane, Cardiff).

Bibliography

Abdel-Khalek, Richardson J. Retinal macroaneurysm: natural history and guidelines for treatment. *Br J Ophthalmol* 1986;**70**:2–11.

Archer DB, Amoaku WMK, Gardiner TA. Radiation retinopathy—Clinical, histopathological, ultrastructural and experimental correlations. *Eye* 1991;**5**:239–51.

Asdourian GK, Golberg MF, Jampol L, Rabb M. Retinal macroaneurysms. *Arch Ophthalmol* 1977;**95**:624–5.

Branch Vein Occlusion Study Group. Argon laser photocoagulation for macular oedema in branch vein occlusion. *Am J Ophthalmol* 1984;**98**:271–82.

Branch Vein Occlusion Study Group. Argon laser photocoagulation for macular oedema in branch vein occlusion. *Am J Ophthalmol* 1985;**99**:218–19.

Branch Vein Occlusion Study Group. Argon scatter photocoagulation for prevention of neovascularisation and vitreous haemorrhage in branch vein occlusion. *Arch Ophthalmol* 1986;**104**:34–41.

Carney MD, Jampol LM. Epiretinal membranes in sickle cell retinopathy. *Arch Ophthalmol* 1987;**105**:214–17.

Casswell AG, Chaine G, Rush P, Bird AC. Paramacular telangiectasia. *Trans Ophthalmol Soc UK* 1986;**105**:63.

Cleary PE, Kohner EM, Hamilton AM, Bird AC. Retinal macroaneurysms. *Br J Ophthalmol* 1975 **59**:355–61.

Cohen SB, Kaplan GR. Sickle cell disease. In: Gold DH, Weingeist TA, eds. *The eye in systemic disease*. Philadelphia: JB Lippincott, 1990; Chapter 50.

Dollery CT, Hodge JV. Hypertensive retinopathy studied with fluorescein. *Trans Ophthalmol Soc UK* 1963;**83**:115–32.

Early Treatment Diabetic Retinopathy Study (ETDRS) Group. Photocoagulation for diabetic macular oedema. Early Treatment Diabetic Study report No 1. *Arch Ophthalmol* 1985;**103**:1796–1806.

Farber MD, Jampol LM, Fox P *et al.* A randomised clinical trial of scatter photocoagulation of proliferative sickle cell retinopathy. *Arch Ophthalmol* 1991;**109**:363–7.

Ferry AP, Combs JL. Wyburn–Mason disease. In: Ryan SJ, ed. *Retina*. St Louis: Mosby, 1989;584–7.

Finkelstein D. Argon laser photocoagulation for macular oedema in branch vein occlusion. *Ophthalmology* 1986;**93**:975–7.

Gagliano DA, Goldberg MF. The evolution of salmon-patch haemorrhages in sickle-cell retinopathy. *Arch Ophthalmol* 1988;**107**:1814–5.

Gass JDM. A fluorescein angiographic study of macular dysfunction secondary to retinal vascular disease. *Arch Ophthalmol* 1968;**80**:535–617.

Gass JDM. *Stereoscopic Atlas of Macular Diseases*. St Louis: Mosby, 1987; Chapter 6. Macular dysfunction caused by retinal vascular disorders.

Gass JD, Oyakawa RT. Idiopathic juxtafoveolar retinal telangiectasia. *Arch Ophthalmol* 1982;**100**:769.

Goldberg MF. Classification and pathogenesis of proliferative sickle retinopathy. *Am J Ophthalmol* 1971;**71**:649–65.

Hamilton AMP, Polkinghorne PJ. Management of diabetic retinopathy. In: Easty DL, ed. *Current ophthalmic surgery*. London: Baillière Tindall, 1990; Chapter 49.

Hayreh SS. Recent advances in fluorescein fundus angiography. *Br J Ophthalmol* 1974;**58**:391–412.

Hayreh SS, Rojas P, Podhajsky P, Montague P, Woolson RF. Ocular neovascularisation with retinal vein occlusion. III: Incidence of ocular neovascularisation with retinal vein occlusion. *Ophthalmology* 1983. **90**:488–506.

Kohner EM, Dollery CT. Fluorescein angiography of the fundus in diabetic retinopathy. *Br Med Bull* 1970;**26**:166–170.

Laatikainen L, Blach RK. Behaviour of the iris vasculature in central retinal vein occlusion: a fluorescein angiographic study of the vascular response of the retina and iris. *Br J Ophthalmol* 1977;**61**:272–7.

Laatikainen L, Kohner EM, Khoury D, Blach RK. Panretinal photocoagulation in central retinal vein occlusion: a randomised controlled study. *Br J Ophthalmol* 1977;**61**:741–53.

Magargal LE, Brown GC, Augsburger JJ, Parish RK. Neovascular glaucoma following central retinal vein occlusion. *Ophthalmology* 1981;**88**:1095.

Mansour AM, Wells CG, Jampol LM, Kalina RE. Ocular complications of arteriovenous communications of the retina. *Arch Ophthalmol* 1981;**107**:232–6.

Maumenee AE. Fluorescein angiography in the diagnosis and treatment of lesions of the ocular fundus. *Trans Ophthalmol Soc UK* 1968;**88**:529–56.

Moriarty BJ, Webb DK, Serjeant GR. Treatment of subretinal neovascularisation associated with angioid streaks in sickle cell retinopathy. *Arch Ophthalmol* 1987;**105**:1327–8 (letter).

Nicholson DM. Capillary hemangioma of the retina and von Hippel–Lindau disease. In: Ryan SJ, ed. *Retina*. St Louis: Mosby, 1989; Chapter 29.

Norton EWD, Gutman F. Diabetic retinopathy studied by fluorescein angiography. *Ophthalmologica* 1965;**150**:5–17.

Ridley ME, Shields JA, Brown GC, Tasman W. Coats' disease. Evaluation of management. *Ophthalmology* 1982;**89**:1381.

Ryan SJ, ed. *Retina*. St Louis: Mosby, 1989;**2(5)**:70–559 (Retinal vascular disease).

Sanborne GE, Magargal LE and Jaeger EA. Venous occlusive disease of the retina. In: Duane TD, ed. *Clinical Ophthalmology*. Town: Harper and Row, 1987: Vol 3, Chapter 15.

Scott DJ, Dollery CT, Hill DW. Fluorescein studies of the retinal circulation in diabetics. *Br J Ophthalmol* 1963;**47**:588–9

Shilling JS and Jones CA. Retinal branch vein occlusion: a study of argon laser photocoagulation in the treatment of macular oedema. *Br J Ophthalmol* 1984;**68**:196–8.

Tso MO. Pathophysiology of hypertensive retinopathy. *Ophthalmology* 1982;**89**:1132–48.

de Venecia G, Davis M, Engerman R. Clinicopathologic correlations in diabetic retinopathy: 1. Histology and fluorescein angiography of microaneurysms. *Arch Ophthalmol* 1976;**94**:1766–73.

Whitelocke RA, Kearns H, Blach RK, Hamilton AM. The diabetic maculopathies. *Trans Ophthalmol Soc UK* 1979;**99**:314–19.

5 Cystoid macular oedema

Many conditions which give rise to increased permeability of the parafoveal capillaries result in cystoid macular oedema (**53**). Fluid collects in the outer plexiform and inner nuclear layers of the retina, forming cystoid spaces in a characteristic pattern. Sometimes these appearances are quite obvious clinically, but on occasions they may be less easy to detect, particularly in the presence of vitritis or opacities of the ocular media. It has been shown that cystoid oedema is often detectable by angiography following cataract surgery (particularly intracapsular surgery, or after vitreous loss) even in the presence of normal acuity (**53**). It is therefore important to differentiate between clinically significant and angiographically proven cystoid macular oedema.

The presence of cystoid macular oedema is of important prognostic significance in a number of conditions (**30, 40, 53, 54**). In diabetic maculopathy, for example, there is a poor response to treatment with photocoagulation. In aphakia, however, a spontaneous recovery occurs in most cases.

Indications for angiography

Determining the presence of cystoid macular oedema In the presence of media opacification, or because there is associated or co-existing macular disease, it may be difficult to distinguish cystoid macular oedema clinically. In these cases the characteristic late appearance of the angiogram may be diagnostic.

53a

following surgery	cataract surgery, particularly intracapsular and following vitreous loss capsulotomy penetrating keratoplasty retinal detachment surgery trabeculectomy, particularly with hypotony
vascular occlusions	central retinal vein occlusion branch vein occlusion
capillary disorders	diabetes macular telangiectasia
inflammatory disorders	chronic uveitis pars planitis birdshot chorioretinitis
subretinal fluid	secondary to: choroidal tumours age-related maculopathy
herododystrophic disorders	retinitis pigmentosa familial exudative vitreoretinopathy
toxicity	adrenaline in aphakia nicotinic acid
preretinal membrane contraction	
idiopathy	

53 (**a**) Causes of cystoid macular oedema.

53b,c,d

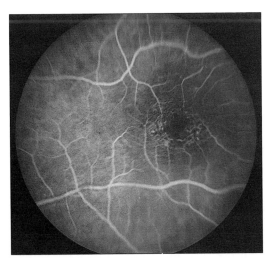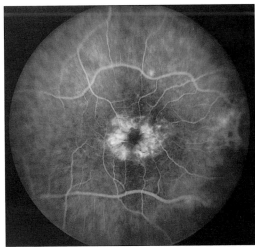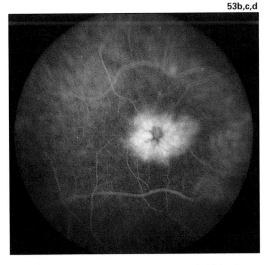

53 Cystoid macular oedema. Cystoid macular oedema following intracapsular cataract extraction. (**b**) Dilated perifoveal capillaries are demonstrated. (**c**) Leakage of dye leads to increasing hyperfluorescence. (**d**) A late photograph shows a petaloid pattern as dye fills the intraretinal cystoid spaces.

Determining the underlying cause If cystoid macular oedema is detected clinically, fluorescein angiography can provide information about the underlying cause. For example, leakage at the disc or other retinal vascular abnormalities may be demonstrated. Angiography is particulary helpful when the primary vascular lesion is long-standing and no longer obvious on biomicroscopy.

Monitoring the effects of treatment Angiography is used to monitor the effect of treatment of cystoid macular oedema, for example acetazolamide in retinitis pigmentosa, steroids in uveitis or vitrectomy to release vitreous traction.

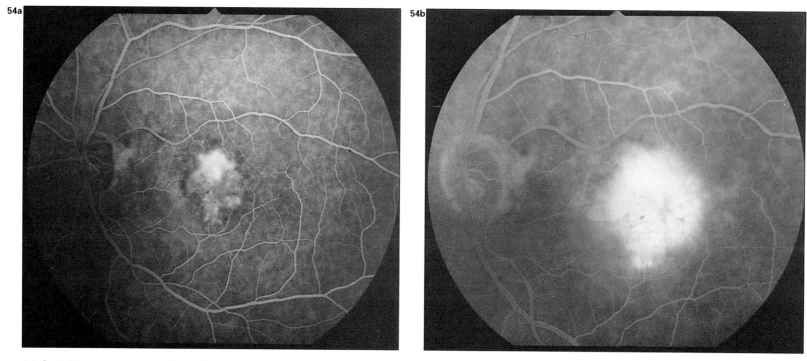

54 Cystoid macular oedema. Cystoid macular oedema associated with age-related choroidal neovascularisation. (**a**) A subretinal neovascular network. (**b**) Late picture demonstrates extensive overlying cystoid oedema.

Bibliography

Fishman GA, Fishman M, Maggiano G. Macular lesions associated with retinitis pigmentosa. *Arch Ophthalmol* 1977; **95**:798–803.

Fung WE. Aphakic cystoid macular edema. In: Ryan SJ. *Retina*, Vol 2. St Louis: Mosby, 1989; Chapter 111.

Fung WE. Other causes of cystoid macular edema. In: Ryan SJ. *Retina*, Vol 2. St Louis: Mosby, 1989; Chapter 112.

Gass JDM, Anderson DR, Davis EB. A clinical, fluorescein angiographic and electron microscopic correlation of cystoid macular oedema. *Am J Ophthalmol* 1985;**100**:82–6.

Gass JDM, Norton EWD. Cystoid macular edema and papilledema following cataract extraction: a fluorescein fundoscopic and angiographic study. *Arch Ophthalmol* 1966;**76**:646–61.

Tso MOM. Pathology of cystoid macular edema. *Ophthalmology* 1982;**89**:902–15.

6 Acquired macular disorders

Age-related maculopathy

This condition has produced a demand for angiography, as an accumulation of evidence has shown the effectiveness of photocoagulation in selected cases. It is important to know the limitations of treatment, to understand clinical appearances and to select cases for angiography that are likely to benefit from treatment. Interpretation of angiograms in age-related maculopathy can sometimes be difficult, even for those with extensive experience. Guidelines for treatment have been derived from large trials with strict entry requirements and the results cannot be applied to cases which do not fulfil these criteria. However, those with experience in the field may treat individual lesions on their merit, and new approaches are continually evolving.

Age-related maculopathy is divided into atrophic and exudative forms. The distinction is useful because at present there is no treatment for the atrophic form, whereas laser photocoagulation may modify the course of some forms of exudative age-related maculopathy.

Atrophic age-related maculopathy

In atrophic age-related maculopathy, there are drusen (**55**) and areas of pigment epithelial atrophy with adjacent pigment clumping

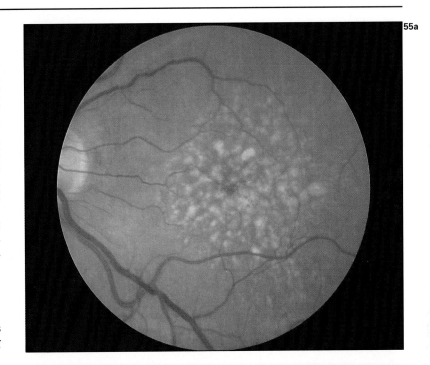

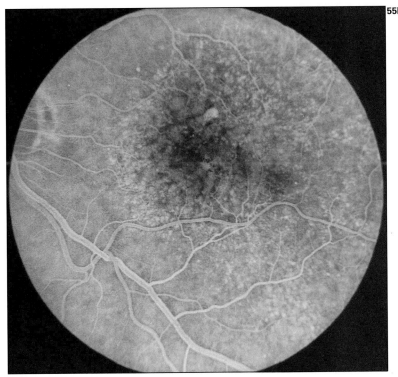

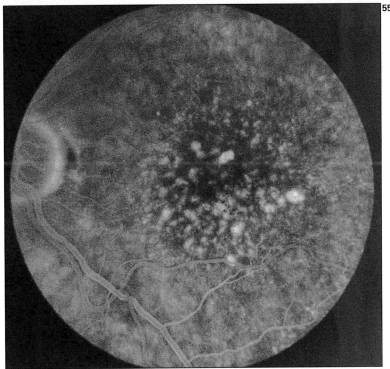

55 Atrophic age-related maculopathy. (**a**) A 64-year-old woman was referred for assessment of her macular appearance. She was asymptomatic with a visual acuity of 6/6 in each eye. (**b**) There is a mixture of small and larger drusen which exhibit hyperfluorescence. Further irregular areas of hyperfluorescence correspond to areas of retinal pigment epithelial atrophy (window or transmission defect, see p. 19). Areas of increased pigmentation correspond to areas of hypofluorescence (blockage, masking, see p. 20). (**c**) The larger central drusen have absorbed fluorescein and continue to fluoresce after the dye has passed through. The smaller, more peripheral drusen are less noticeable in this frame.

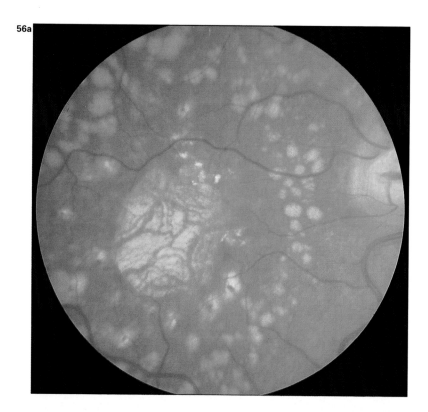

(55,56,57). The atrophic areas may progress to full-thickness confluent atrophy, with well-defined borders in a 'geographic' pattern. No fluid is present beneath the retina or pigment epithelium. Visual loss may be gradual and it is often difficult to predict the visual acuity from the clinical appearances, although if a patch of geographic atrophy affects the central fovea, acuity is usually poor.

Drusen are common in the aging fundus. They are yellowish deposits of extracellular material under the pigment epithelium, ranging in shape and size from small, well-defined round structures ('hard' drusen) to larger and more irregular lesions which appear to coalesce ('soft' drusen). Some develop a sparkling, crystalline appearance. The pattern of drusen distribution is very variable but is often symmetrical in the two eyes. Although usually most prominent in the macular area, they sometimes extend to surround the disc and into the midperiphery of the fundus.

Angiographic appearances

Drusen These structures fluoresce on angiography, and the intensity of fluorescence depends on a combination of transmission defect and absorption of dye (55,56,57,66). Angiography often reveals greater numbers than can be detected on biomicroscopy. Most drusen fluoresce early because of defects in the overlying pigment epithelium. In general, the hyperfluorescent area remains constant in shape and size. The absorption of dye and the persistence of hyperfluorescence

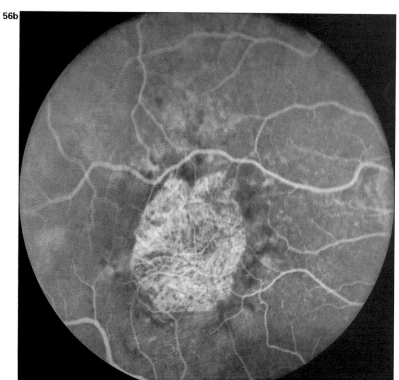

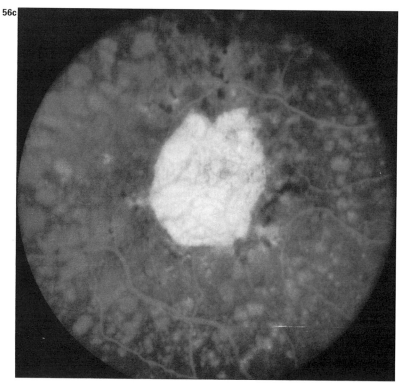

56 Atrophic age-related maculopathy – geographic atrophy. (a) A 68-year-old woman had noticed a gradual deterioration of vision. Visual acuity was 6/60 in each eye. (b,c) There is a pattern of 'soft' drusen which are not prominent in (b) but which remain hyperfluorescent in the late phase. There is a sharply demarcated area of geographic atrophy in each eye. Larger choroidal vessels are visible, indicating loss of the overlying pigment epithelium and choriocapillaris. There is intense late hyperfluorescence but no evidence of spread beyond the boundaries of the atrophic area, demonstrating a transmission defect with no evidence of breakdown of the outer blood–retinal barrier. Note the absence of drusen in the atrophic area.

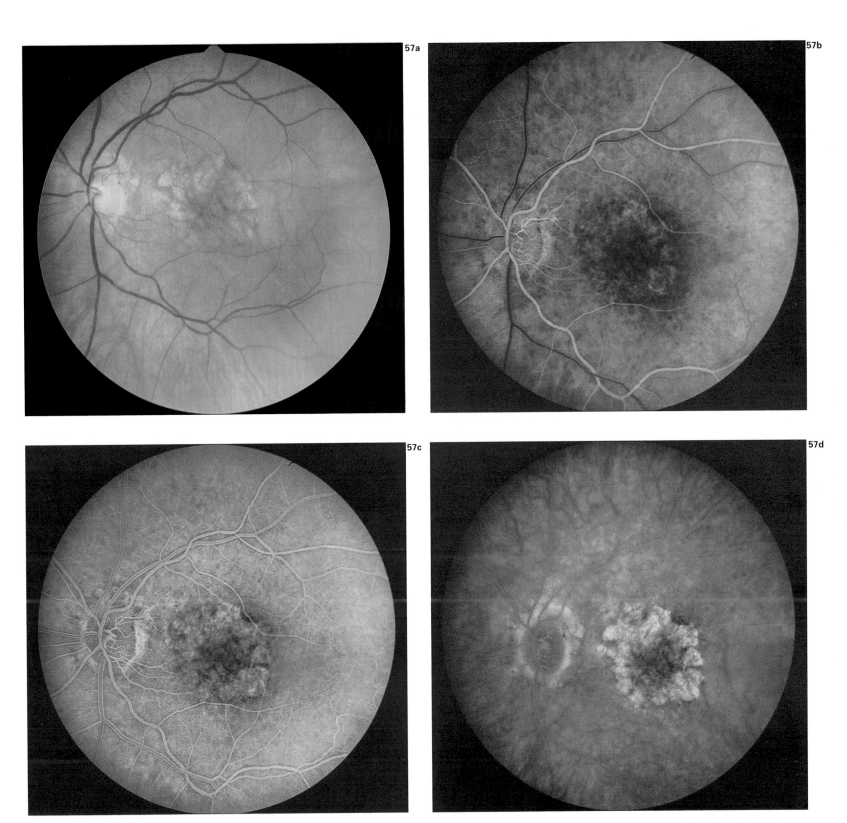

57 Atrophic age-related maculopathy. (**a,b,c,d**) A 76-year-old man had noticed increasing difficulty reading. Visual acuity was 6/9, N5; 6/9, N12. The right eye showed pigment epithelial atrophy. There was early geographic atrophy with central sparing on the left.

depend on their structure. With some drusen the fluorescence fades as the dye leaves the choroid, whereas with others, notably the larger soft drusen, fluorescence persists as dye stains the deposit.

Retinal pigment epithelial atrophy and pigment clumping These phenomena are seen as 'window' defects and masking, respectively (**55,56,57**).

Geographic atrophy appears as well-defined areas of hyperfluorescence, resulting from atrophy of the pigment epithelium and eventual disappearance of the choriocapillaris (**56,57**). In the absence of the choriocapillaris, the large choroidal vessels are visible as they fill with dye in the early part of the angiogram, and later appear as hypofluorescent streaks against the background of the staining of the sclera.

Indications for angiography

In the absence of subretinal fluid there is no point in performing angiography, as no form of treatment has yet been shown to influence the course of the disease. If there is an element of doubt about the presence of subretinal fluid, fluorescein angiography may be helpful.

Exudative age-related maculopathy

In contrast to atrophic maculopathy, the onset of exudative age-related maculopathy is usually rapid. The patient notices a deterioration in central acuity, often accompanied by distortion. Frequently, however, patients are unaware of problems with one eye until the vision is grossly impaired, or until the other becomes affected. Fundus examination shows the presence of subretinal fluid with varying degrees of haemorrhage and exudate. The red or greyish outline of a subretinal network is sometimes visible, but more often it is obscured by overlying fluid and haemorrhage. Signs of atrophic maculopathy are usually present to some degree and, if extensive, may make clinical assessment difficult.

There is still discussion about the exact pathological processes producing the various clinical pictures seen in exudative age-related maculopathies, but it is convenient to classify them on the basis of angiographic appearances as this provides a guide to management:

- Subretinal neovascularization:
  discrete, well-defined;
  obscured;
  occult.
- Pigment epithelial detachment

Angiographic appearances

In the presence of lens opacities in the elderly, angiographic appearances may be difficult to interpret. Nevertheless, it is usually possible to decide whether the lesion is treatable even though a detailed analysis may not be feasible. Stereoscopic angiography is of considerable benefit in many cases, giving information about retinal thickness and elevation. Misinterpretation is possible if angiograms are examined in isolation. Colour pictures are often of poor quality in this age group and in some cases is it difficult to make an accurate assessment without re-examining the patient.

Choroidal neovascularization It is now generally agreed that where there is a well-defined subretinal neovascular network eccentric to the fovea, laser treatment should be considered as long as it is possible to obliterate completely the network without threatening central acuity. Angiography is a prerequisite when laser treatment is being contemplated to identify the membrane, to assess its extent and to determine the foveal centre (**58,59,60,61,62**).

A well-defined neovascular membrane appears early in the angiogram as the fine new vessels fill from the choroid (**58,59**). The membrane then becomes more intensely fluorescent, with spread of fluorescence beyond its margins as dye leaks out during the following 1–2 minutes, eventually spreading throughout the subretinal fluid. Sometimes the delicate frond of new vessels is clearly visible, but often the rapid leakage of dye and the poor quality of the image make this difficult to detect. The network can nevertheless be identified in later frames by its intense fluorescence, often more marked near its margins, and by evidence of leakage. Size varies from a small dot to a large area occupying most of the macular area. The edges are characteristically irregular, but symmetrical, circular lesions are seen occasionally.

In some cases the neovascular complex is ill-defined, with borders partly obscured by haemorrhage or pigment. Angiography in these circumstances fails to demonstrate the whole extent of the complex.

58a

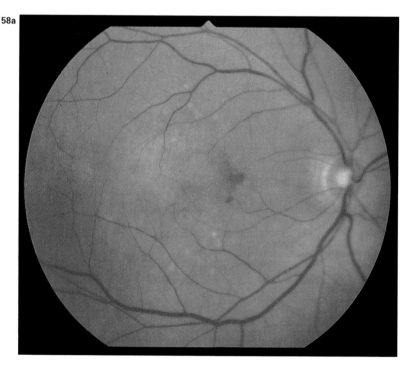

58 Subretinal neovascular network. (**a**) A 71-year-old man noticed a shadow over his right eye. His visual acuity was 6/24. A fluorescein angiogram performed at this stage was unhelpful because a large haemorrhage obscured the underlying neovascular network. Another angiogram was performed when the haemorrhage cleared.

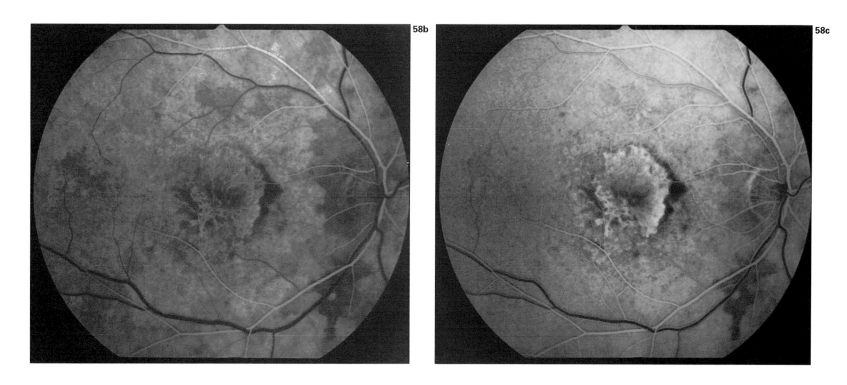

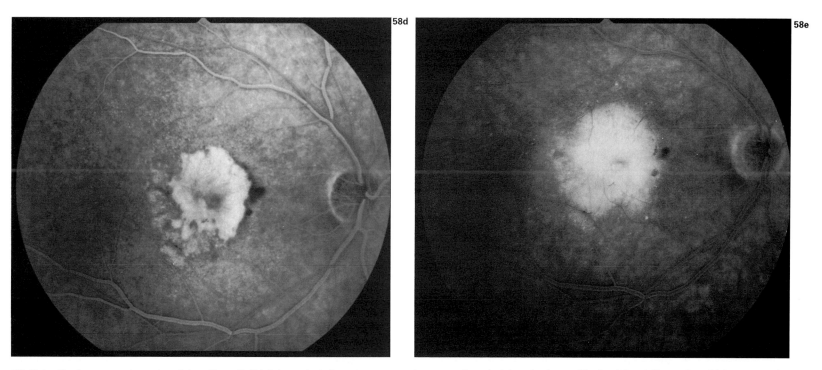

58 Subretinal neovascular network (continued). (**b**) A large but discrete neovascular network underlying the fovea. Much of the delicate choroidal neovascular frond is clearly defined. (**c,d**) The hyperfluorescence becomes more intense and confluent as dye leaks from the new vessels.(**e**) The hyperfluorescence clearly extends beyond the boundaries of the neovascular frond as dye fills the subretinal space.

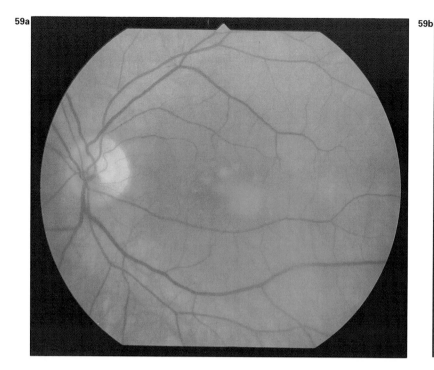

59a

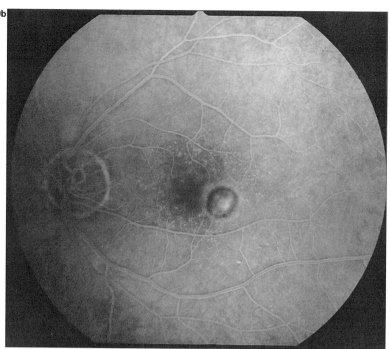

59b

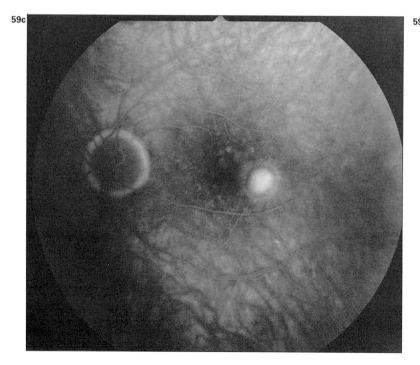

59c

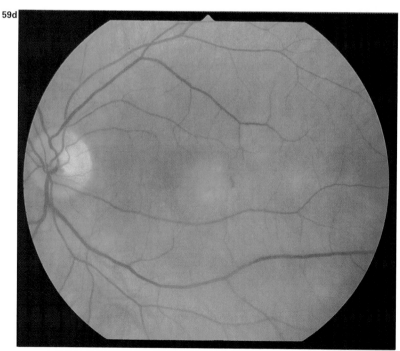

59d

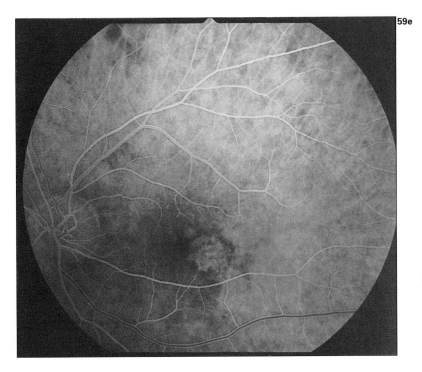

59e

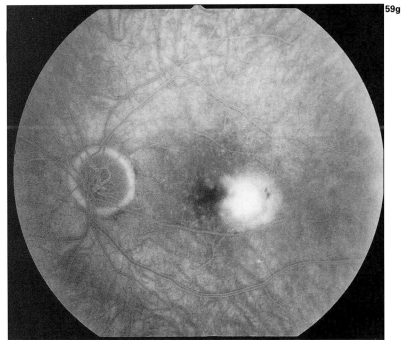

59g

59 Subretinal neovascular network. (a) A 68-year-old man complained of distortion, and had a visual acuity of 6/9. (b,c) An angiogram demonstrates a discrete hyperfluorescent lesion. (d) Fundus appearance six months later. (e,f,g) Six months later, the lesion has shown typical growth and demonstrates all the features of a discrete neovascular network. It is no longer possible to treat without threatening central acuity. Visual acuity had fallen to 2/60 six months later.

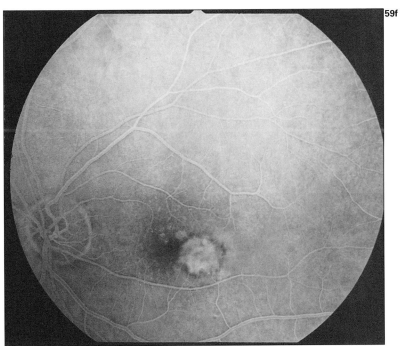

59f

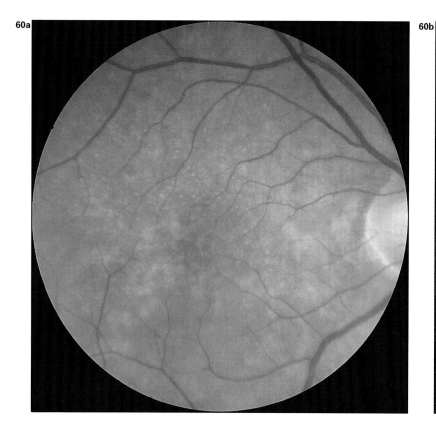

60a

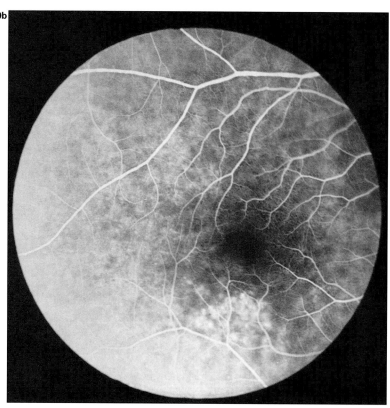

60b

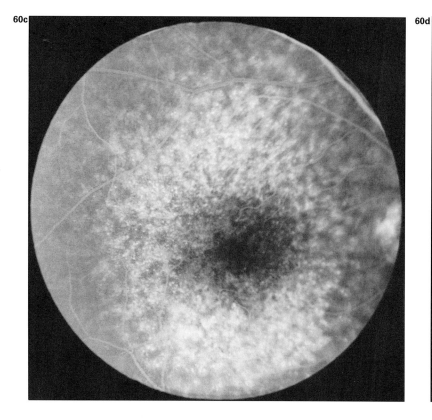

60c

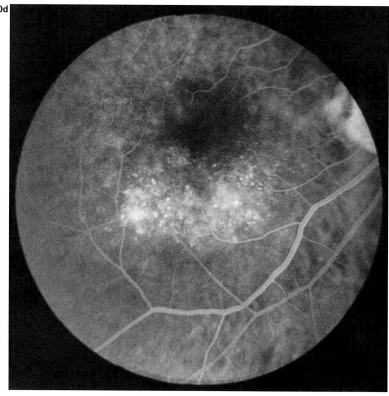

60d

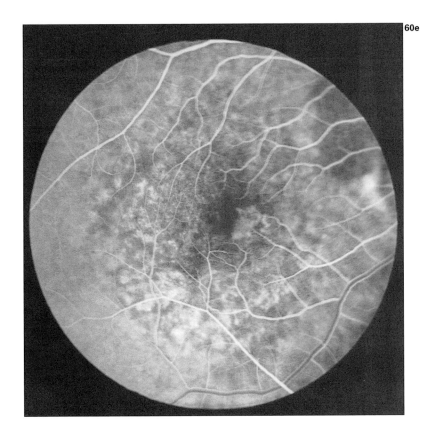

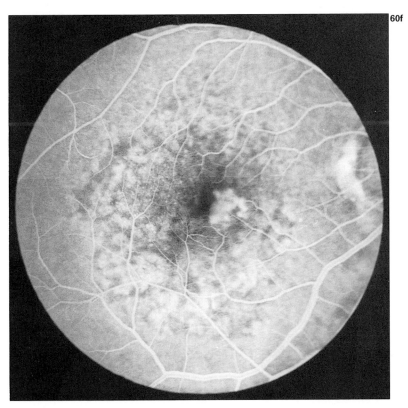

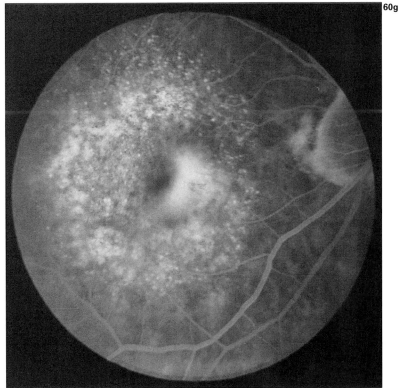

60 Exudative age-related maculopathy. (**a**) An elderly woman complained of progressive deterioration of her central vision with distortion. An area of subretinal fluid was present inferior to the right fovea. (**b**) A patch of hyperfluorescence is seen below the fovea. (**c**) There is more widespread fluorescence as numerous drusen become apparent. The patch noted in (**b**) is no longer prominent. (**d**) As fluorescence fades, the area first seen in (**b**) again stands out. There is diffuse spread of dye between the small hyperfluorescent foci. Occult new vessels are suspected. (**e,f,g**) A year later, there is a discrete neovascular membrane in an unrelated area. The pattern of hyperfluorescence over the rest of the macula, however, shows that a more widespread exudative process coexists.

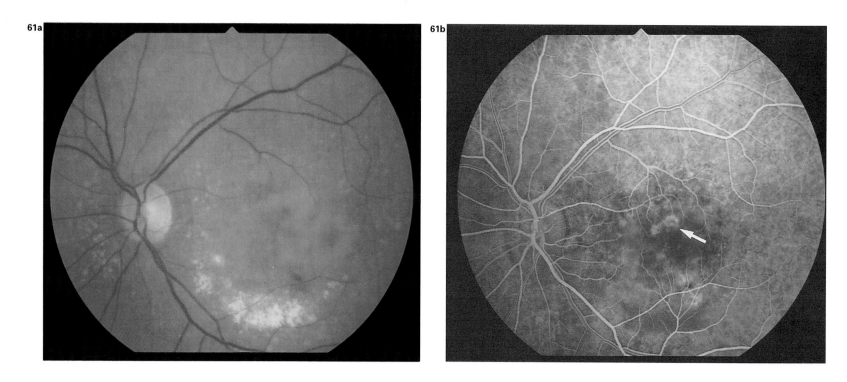

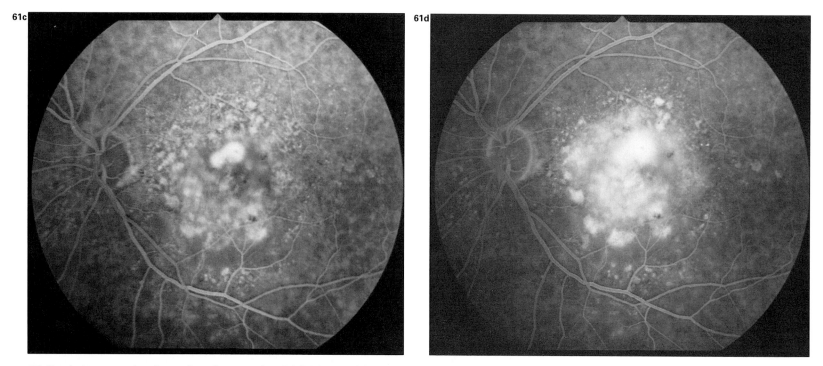

61 Exudative age-related maculopathy: complex. (**a**) A 72-year-old man had poor vision in both eyes, but over the past three weeks had noticed a further deterioration in the left. At the left macula were subretinal fluid, haemorrhage and exudate. (**b**) There are foci of hyperfluorescence, and one area is reasonably well defined (arrow).(**c,d**) The defined area becomes increasingly fluorescent with the leakage of dye, but it becomes clear that there are many other foci of leakage and there is little doubt that there is extensive underlying neovascularization.

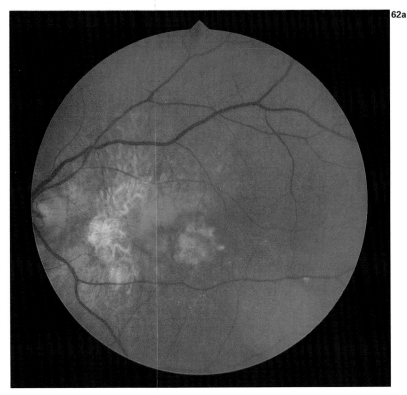

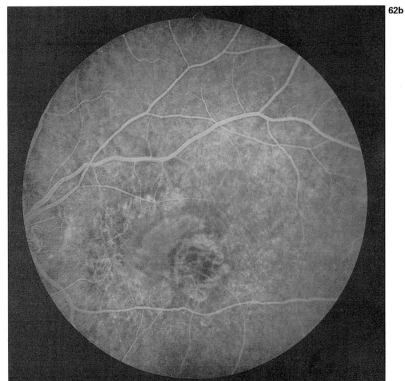

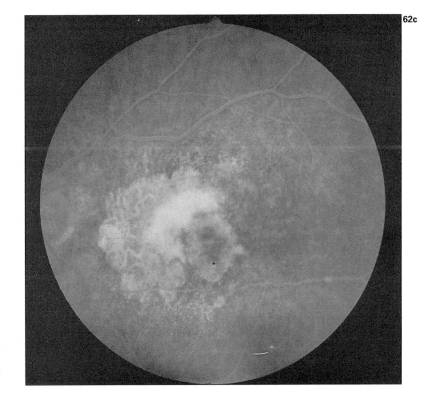

62 Recurrent subretinal neovascularization. A 77-year-old man noticed distortion in his left eye. He had a disciform scar in his right eye and had been warned to attend casualty at the first sign of symptoms on the left. The visual acuity at presentation was 6/6. A small eccentric neovascular membrane was treated. For the next 14 months he maintained a visual acuity of 6/9, but then noticed a sudden deterioration of his vision. (**a**) A grey elevated patch lies adjacent to the treatment scar. (**b**) Angiography demonstrates recurrent neovascularization at the foveal edge of the laser scar with leakage on the late picture. (**c**) The well-defined area of hyperfluorescence between the neovascular network and the disc corresponds to an atrophic area on the colour picture.

In some cases there is biomicroscopic evidence of subretinal fluid or exudation, but no discrete, well-defined neovascular network or obvious pigment epithelial detachment. Angiography demonstrates an ill-defined leakage, which may be diffuse and widespread or more localized. Often, patches of small hyperfluorescent spots become increasingly fluorescent, giving a late diffuse hyperfluorescence. In these cases either there are occult new vessels present, or the outer blood–retinal barrier is chronically disrupted (**60,61**).

Pigment epithelial detachments Pigment epithelial detachments are usually diagnosed clinically by biomicroscopy, but can sometimes be difficult to detect when retinal elevation is slight and no fluid is present between the pigment epithelium and neuroretina. Fluorescein angiography is helpful in establishing the diagnosis and assessing whether any neovascularization is present (**63,64,65,66,67**).

Pigment epithelial detachments demonstrate a characteristic homogeneous fluorescence which does not change in shape or size during the course of the angiogram, although its intensity alters (**64,65**). There are variations in the rate at which pigment epithelial detachments fill, and the pattern of fill may be regular or irregular. The presence of blood, irregular edges and foci of more intense fluorescence suggest the existence of neovascularization within the lesion (**65**). Occasionally, either spontaneously or following photocoagula-

tion, a rip may develop at one edge of a pigment epithelial detachment giving a characteristic clinical picture (**67**). The torn edge contracts leaving a semilunar, sharp-edged pigmented area and a corresponding exposed area of choroid. Central vision is markedly impaired in such cases.

Angiography is mainly of diagnostic use in the management of pigment epithelial detachments, as the results of laser treatment have been found to be disappointing. Even if successful flattening of the elevated pigment epithelium is produced, subsequent atrophy often leads to further visual loss. There is no evidence to date that some types of pigment epithelial detachments respond better to laser treatment than others.

Determination of the foveal centre The exact position of the foveal avascular zone and the foveal centre—important landmarks if treatment is being contemplated—is sometimes difficult to determine. A fixation target which appears on the developed film can be helpful, but may be misleading where central fixation is impaired. A useful approach is to project the frames which show the best view of the macular vessels, and to trace those which are distinguishable on to a piece of paper. Even when the vessels are not visible as far as the capillary free zone, the pattern they form gives a valuable clue to the position of the fovea.

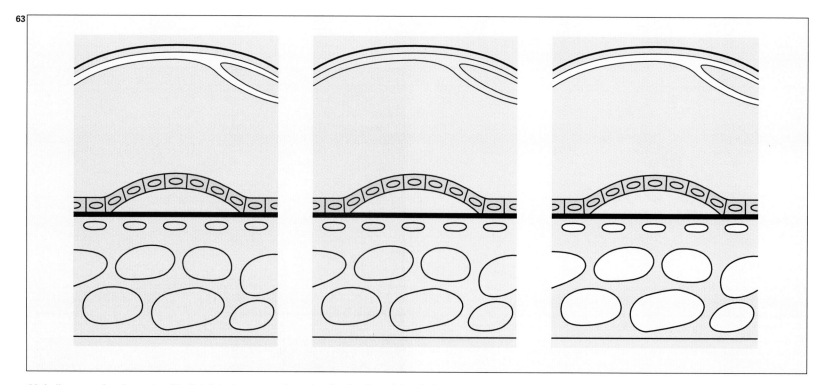

63 A diagram of a pigment epithelial detachment to show the distribution of dye during the course of an angiogram.

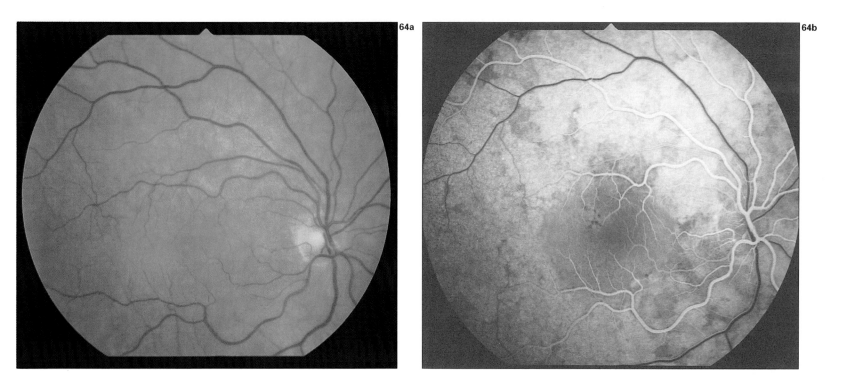

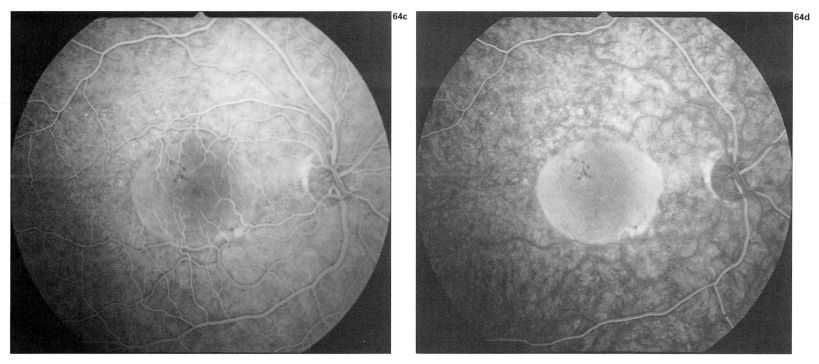

64 Pigment epithelial detachment – even filling. A 63-year-old woman complained of distortion and reduced visual acuity (6/24) in the right eye. She had a disciform scar in the other eye. (**a**) The colour photograph demonstrates how difficult it can sometimes be to detect a pigment epithelial detachment clinically without a binocular view.(**b**) The pigment epithelial detachment masks underlying choroidal fluorescence while showing early fluorescence itself. (**c**) The margins of the detachment are now defined. (**d**) The lesion becomes more intensely fluorescent during the course of the angiogram and remains hyperfluorescent as retinal vascular fluorescence fades.

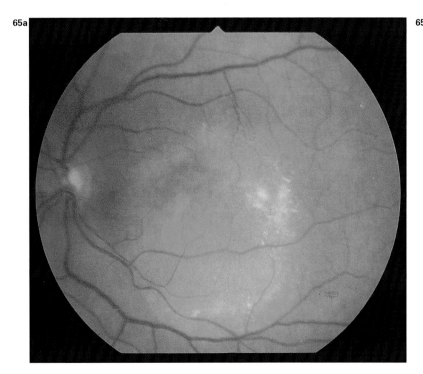

65a

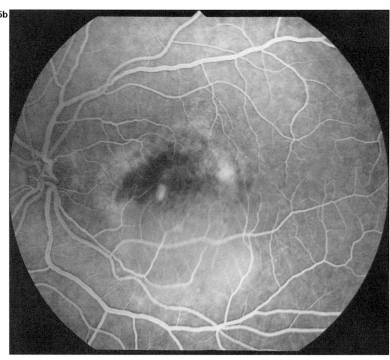

65b

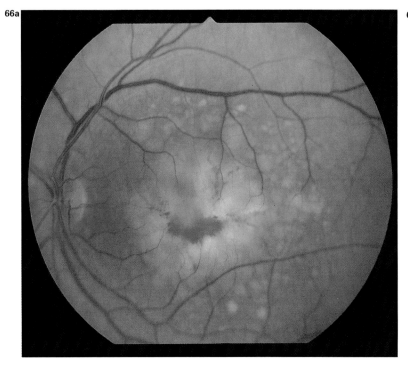

66a

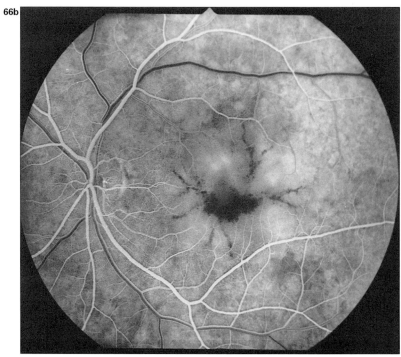

66b

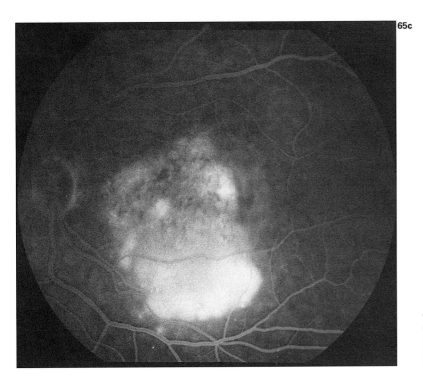

65 Pigment epithelial detachment – irregular filling. A 68-year-old woman complained of distortion in her left eye. Visual acuity was 6/18. (a) A large pigment epithelial detachment with exudates. (b,c) The pigment epithelial detachment is irregular and patches of more intense hyperfluorescence are seen. Neovascularization is strongly suspected.

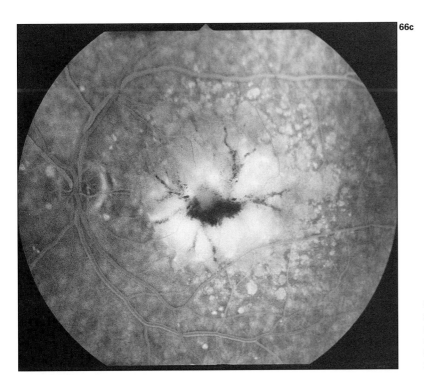

66 Pigment epithelial detachment. (a) An elderly man had suffered a gradual deterioration of his visual acuity (6/24, 6/24). Extensive soft drusen appear to coalesce centrally. A pigment figure overlies the central elevated area. The other eye showed a similar appearance. (b,c) The angiographic appearances are indistinguishable from those of a pigment epithelial detachment. Note masking corresponding to the radiating pattern of pigment.

Indications for angiography

A doubtful diagnosis Exudative age-related maculopathy can be accompanied by marked retinal elevation, exudation, and haemorrhage. The appearances vary considerably and may be confused with those of choroidal tumours and conditions affecting the retinal vasculature, for example macular branch vein occlusions, and macroaneurysms.

A suspected treatable lesion Fluorescein angiography is indicated to determine whether a treatable lesion is present and to delineate its full extent. Subretinal neovascular networks often grow quickly and treatment should be instituted as soon as possible after the onset of symptoms. A lesion is more likely to be amenable to treatment if the visual acuity is good (6/18 or better) and if symptoms have been present for less than a month.

Monitoring treatment Angiography can be used to assess whether a lesion has been successfully treated, and to detect suspected recurrences. For all these situations, the following principles apply:

- Perform angiography as soon as possible, preferably within a few days of onset of symptoms.
- Any treatment should be based on a recent angiogram. Fluorescein angiographic services should be organized to allow rapid access and processing for these cases.
- There is little value in performing angiography if treatment is not contemplated. For example: where the lesion is too large, or obviously subfoveal; where extensive haemorrhage obscures the full extent of the neovascular membrane; where the patient would, for whatever reason, be unable to co-operate with treatment; where media opacities would render treatment impossible; or where the lesion has reached the stage of scarring. If there is any element of doubt, however, especially if this is the second affected eye, angiography should be performed.

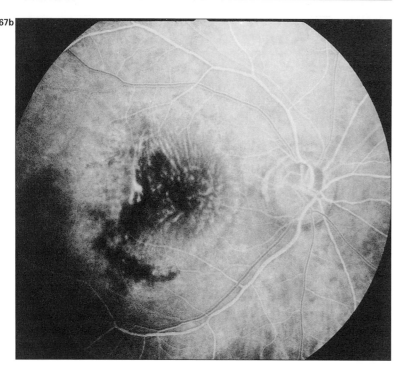

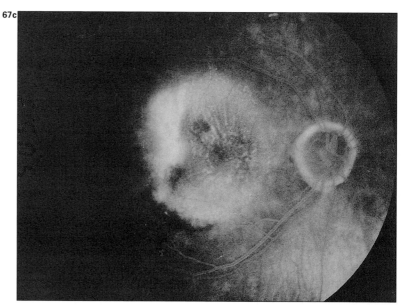

67 Tear of the retinal pigment epithelium. **(a)** A 77-year-old woman noticed a rapid loss of vision in one eye. At the time of the angiogram visual acuity was 6/18, but over the next few months it deteriorated to 6/60. **(b,c)** There has been a spontaneous rip or tear in a pigment epithelial detachment. Lateral to the straight edge of the tear is an area of hyperfluorescence corresponding to exposed choriocapillaris. The surface of the pigment epithelial detachment has a wrinkled appearance and there is probably an associated new vessel membrane.

Other conditions associated with choroidal neovascularization

Almost any fundus condition which causes injury or atrophy of the retinal pigment epithelium or Bruch's membrane may induce secondary choroidal new vessels, particularly in the macular area. In clinical practice some associations are more common than others and only those most frequently encountered are discussed in this section. The primary diagnosis is seldom in doubt and angiography is usually performed in order to determine the presence of neovascularization, to assess whether photocoagulation is indicated, and to monitor the treatment. Some disorders, such as presumed ocular histoplasmosis, have localized retinal pigment epithelial atrophy and laser treatment is normally effective. In those with widespread retinal pigment epithelial changes, such as pseudoxanthoma elasticum, the response to treatment is more unpredictable.

High (degenerative) myopia

Progressive elongation of the eye in high myopia is associated with secondary degenerative changes in the fundus.

Chorioretinal atrophy Thinning of the retinal pigment epithelium and choroid gives rise to a pale appearance with increased visibility of the large choroidal vessels. As the process continues, patches of chorioretinal atrophy develop. The chorioretinal attenuation results in increased transmission of fluorescence from the sclera, reducing contrast on the angiogram. Details of the retinal capillary network are therefore difficult to distinguish, and the centre of the fovea may be difficult to locate (**68**).

Lacquer cracks Breaks in Bruch's membrane give rise to pale, sharp-edged streaks which hyperfluoresce on fluorescein angiography. Adjacent spontaneous haemorrhages often develop but then clear without sequelae. However, cracks are also associated with choroidal neovascularization, which often leads to a permanent reduction in central vision.

Choroidal neovascularization The disciform lesions associated with high myopia, which characteristically give rise to the appearance known as the Foerster–Fuchs spot, have certain features which differ from age-related disease (**69**). They tend to be small and round and often have a pigmented halo. The scar left after resolution is usually small, but many of the lesions are close to the foveal centre and cause significant visual deterioration, though often less severe than with age-related maculopathy. On fluorescein angiography, the leakage from the lesion is more circumscribed than in age-related maculopathy.

Angioid streaks

Angioid streaks are jagged red lines, so-called because their colour, width and radial orientation invites comparison with retinal vessels (**70**). They are cracks in Bruch's membrane and are found in a range of conditions, including pseudoxanthoma elasticum, Paget's disease, fibrodysplasia hyperelastica (Ehlers–Danlos syndrome) and sickle-cell anaemia. Angioid streaks are most commonly detected in pseudoxanthoma elasticum and can be the presenting feature. The streaks fluoresce early and the fluorescence persists into the residual phase. The patient often presents with loss of central vision and a neovascular lesion at, or near, the foveal centre. Results of photocoagulation have been disappointing, though treatment may be beneficial in selected cases.

Idiopathic disciform

Spontaneous choroidal neovascularization occasionally occurs in younger age groups, sometimes as early as the second decade, where there is no other evidence of the changes associated with aging and no other obvious precipitating factor (**71**). Treatment should be considered if central vision is threatened.

Trauma – choroidal tears

Blunt trauma may result in rupture of Bruch's membrane. The retinal pigment epithelium is very rarely torn, but leakage through it is detectable soon after injury (**72**). This tends to resolve, but in cases of tears in the macular area, choroidal new vessels can develop. Fluorescein angiography demonstrates hyperfluorescence corresponding to the pallor seen clinically. As in angioid streaks, the lesion fluoresces early and remains fluorescent in late frames. In the acute phase there may be masking associated with haemorrhage. When ruptures pass close to the fovea, angiography is helpful in delineating suspected areas of secondary choroidal neovascularization.

Presumed ocular histoplasmosis (POHS)

This condition is common in central and eastern USA, where it is thought to be caused by previous infection with the fungus, *Histoplasma capsulatum*. A similar fundus appearance is seen, though much less frequently, in other parts of the world in people who have never travelled to endemic areas. In these cases there is no evidence of infection with histoplasma and the aetiology is unknown. Fundus examination shows peripapillary atrophy of the retinal pigment epithelium and small, well-defined, peripheral atrophic spots or lines (**73**). The patient is usually asymptomatic until a disciform lesion develops from a previous atrophic spot near the fovea.

Peripapillary neovascularization

Peripapillary choroidal new vessels occur in the elderly, but are also occasionally seen in younger age groups. They occur in association with a wide range of conditions which result in peripapillary chorioretinal abnormalities, including all the causes of choroidal neovascularization already mentioned in this chapter. The neovascularization extends from the disc towards the fovea and may be unilateral or bilateral (**74**). The lesion appears to progress at a slower rate than macular new vessels and treatment is often deferred until central acuity is threatened. Angiography shows the usual features of choroidal neovascularization, but arising close to the disc rather than at the macula. In many cases the margins of the lesion are poorly defined or obscured by haemorrhage, and it may be difficult to judge its full extent when treatment is planned.

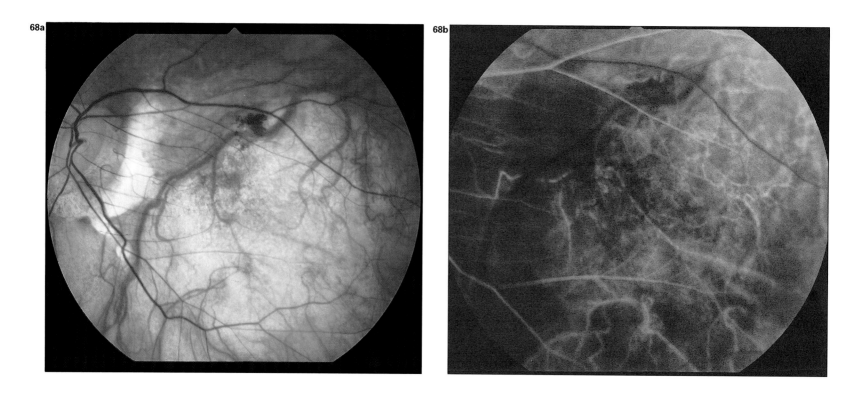

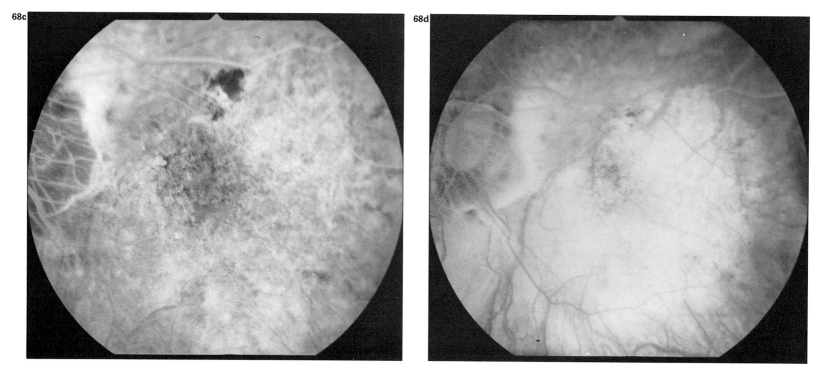

68 Degenerative myopia. (**a**) A 63-year-old woman with degenerative myopia had noticed distortion in her left eye. A small haemorrhage is visible below the upper temporal arcade. The angiogram demonstrates some of the features of a myopic fundus which make interpretation difficult.(**b**) Increased visibility of the choroidal vessels. (**c**) Marked chorioretinal attenuation with increased transmission of fluorescein from the sclera. The resulting hyperfluorescence reduces contrast and no details of the capillary bed are visible. A patch of hypofluorescence confirms that a haemorrhage is present. (**d**) No useful detail is visible against the background hyperfluorescence.

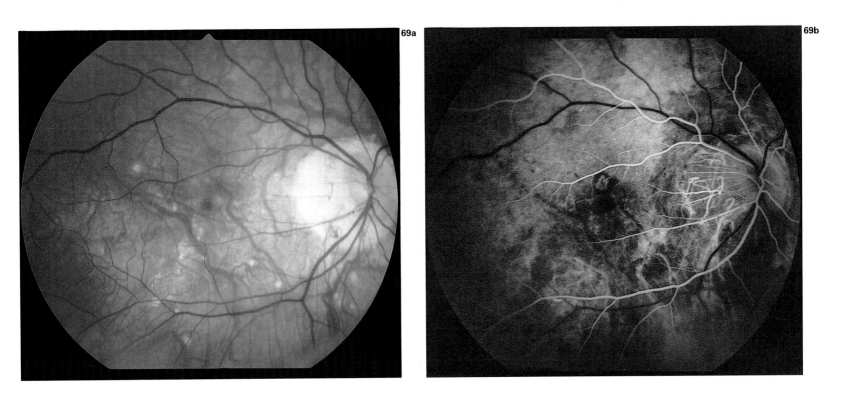

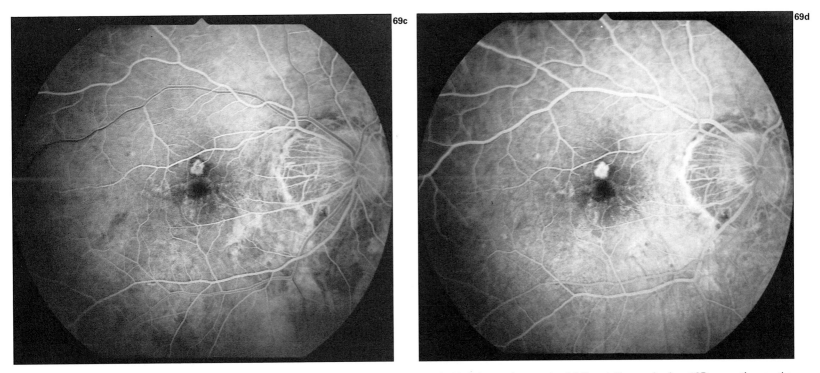

69 Myopia – subretinal neovascular membrane. (**a**) A 43-year-old man had poor vision in his left eye since early childhood. He required a –13D correction on the right. He complained of distortion with his right eye. (**b,c,d**) A small, well-circumscribed neovascular network is demonstrated.

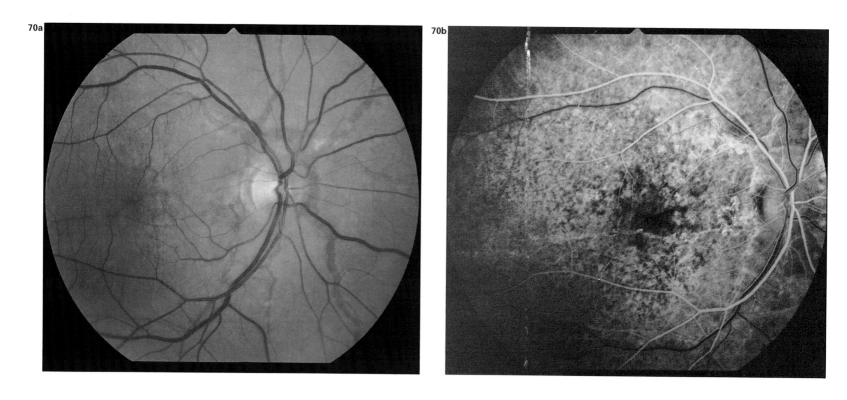

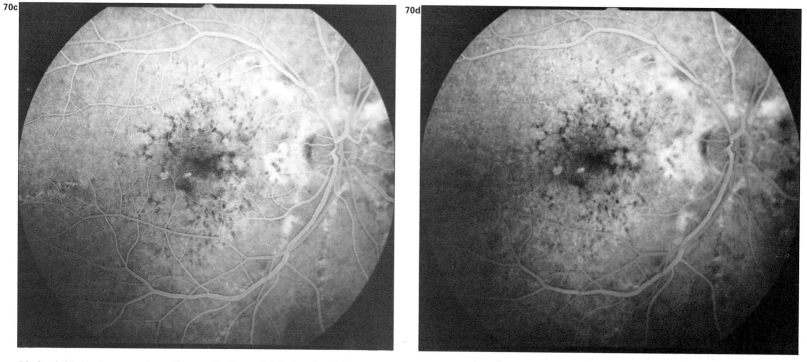

70 Angioid streaks – pseudoxanthoma elasticum. (**a**) At the age of 37 this woman had noticed a sudden blurring of her left vision. She was found to have angioid streaks and a skin biopsy confirmed the presence of pseudoxanthoma elasticum. The left visual acuity eventually deteriorated to 6/60. Nine years later she noticed similar symptoms on the right. (**b**) The streaks show early hyperfluorescence. (**c,d**) Two small discrete hyperfluorescent areas appear along the streak which passes horizontally through the macula, suggesting the presence of early choroidal neovascularization. The patient was treated, but unfortunately her vision continued to deteriorate and stabilized at 6/60 in each eye.

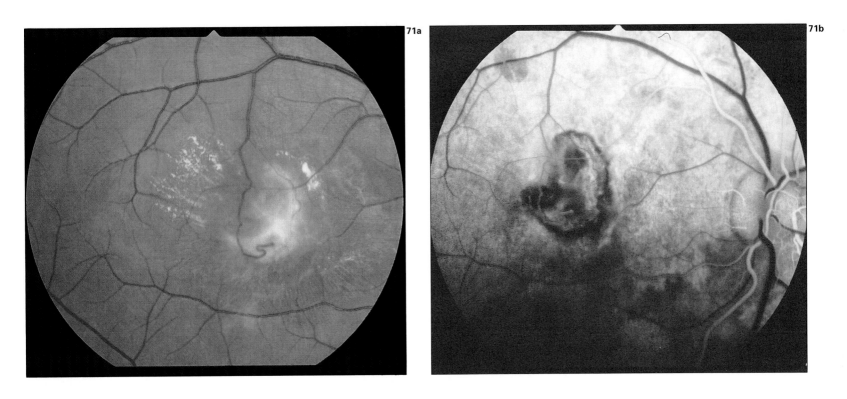

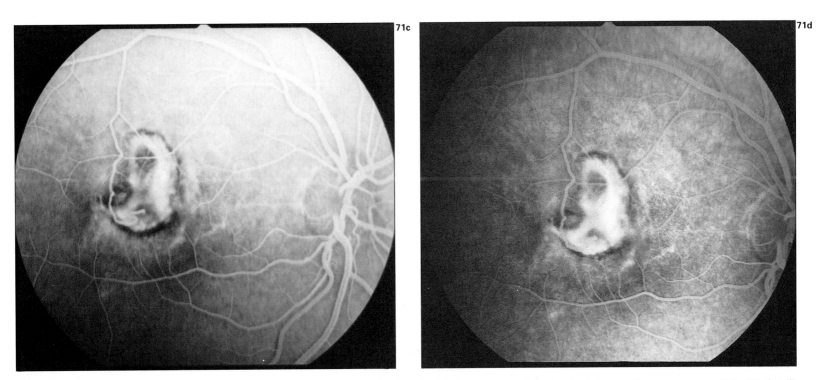

71 Idiopathic choroidal neovascularization. (**a**) A 14-year-old boy had noticed gradual deterioration of vision in his right eye. Visual acuity was 6/60, 6/4. (**b,c,d**) There is a subfoveal neovascular network. A chorioretinal anastomosis is present.

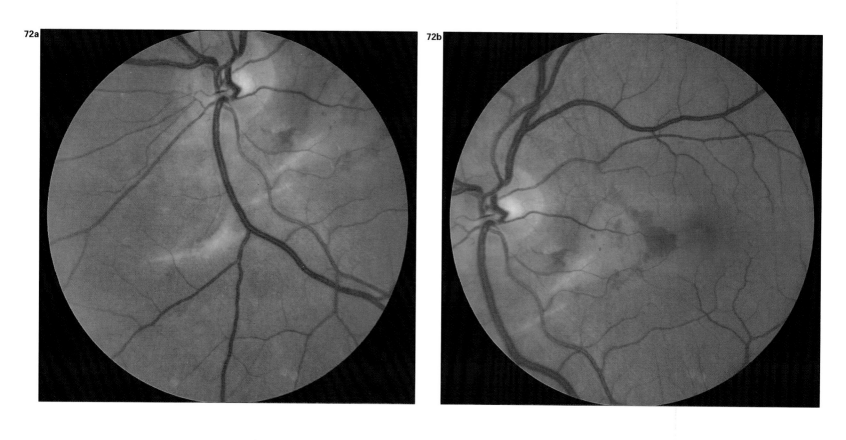

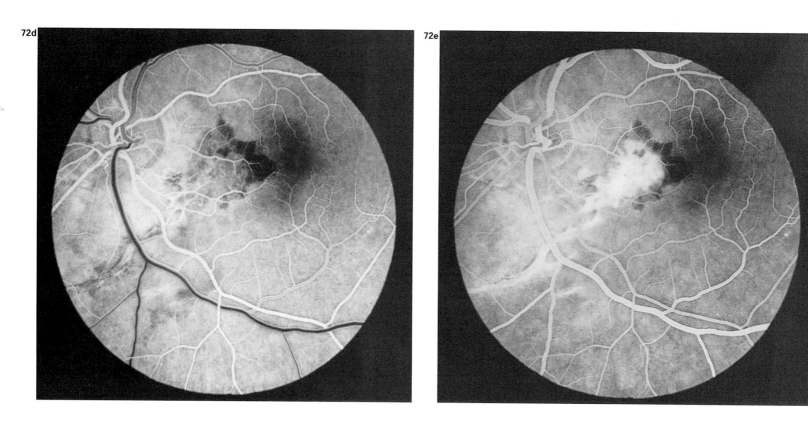

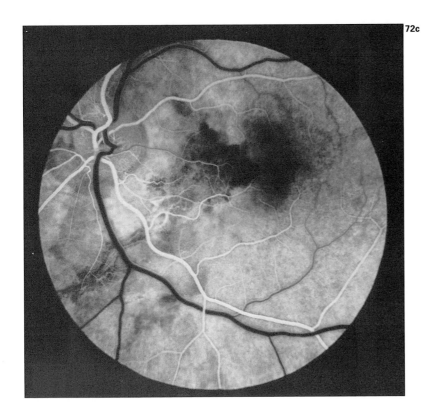

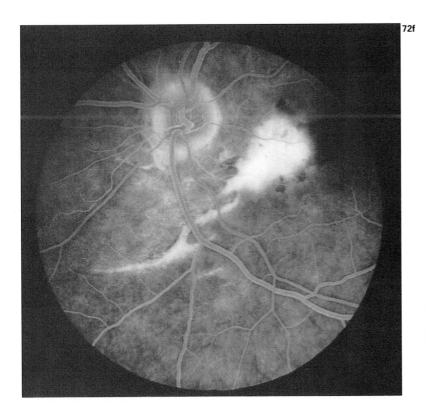

72 Choroidal rupture – secondary neovascular membrane. (**a,b**) A 34-year-old man was assaulted with a blunt object, sustaining zygomatic and nasal fractures. Examination of the eye showed traumatic mydriasis and a choroidal rupture, with a visual acuity of 6/12. Several months later he noticed a sudden drop of visual acuity to less than 6/60 and an angiogram was performed. (**c**) There is early fluorescence along the course of a tear concentric with the disc. (**d,e**) A large neovascular network is present nasal to the fovea. Its full extent is obscured by haemorrhage. (**f**) The late picture shows leakage from the network. Staining of the underlying sclera is visible along the path of the tear. Further smaller concentric tears are also visible.

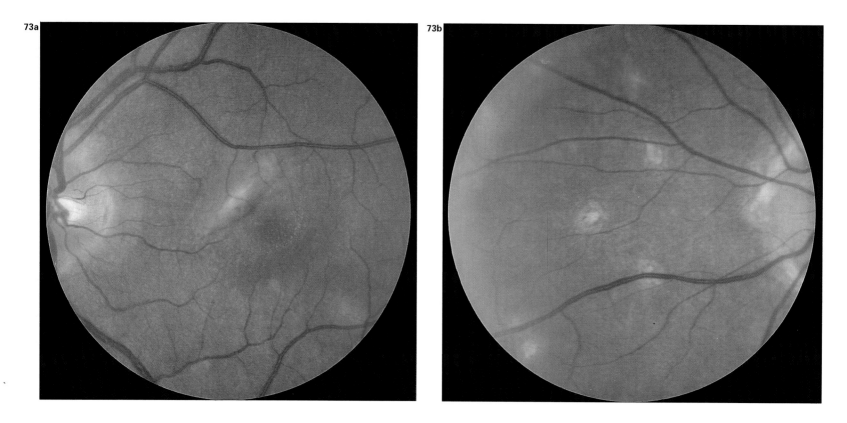

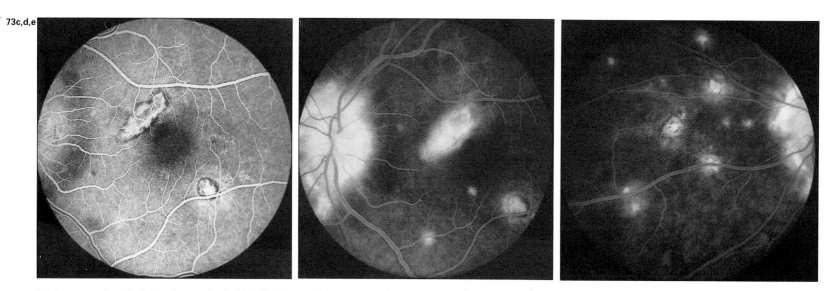

73 Presumed ocular histoplasmosis. (**a,b**) A fit 35-year-old woman woke up one morning to find her vision was blurred. (**c,d**) Two neovascular networks are demonstrated. Two further hyperfluorescent spots correspond with pale areas which are barely perceptible on the colour photograph. Note the hyperfluorescence around the disc. (**e**) The peripheral spots are hyperfluorescent.

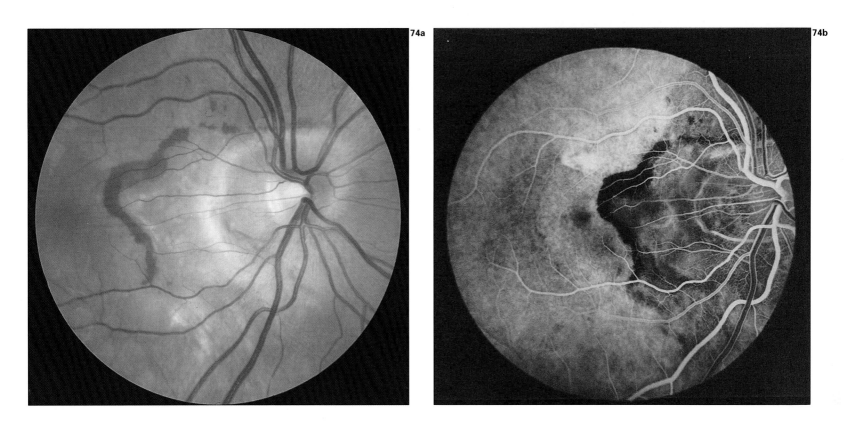

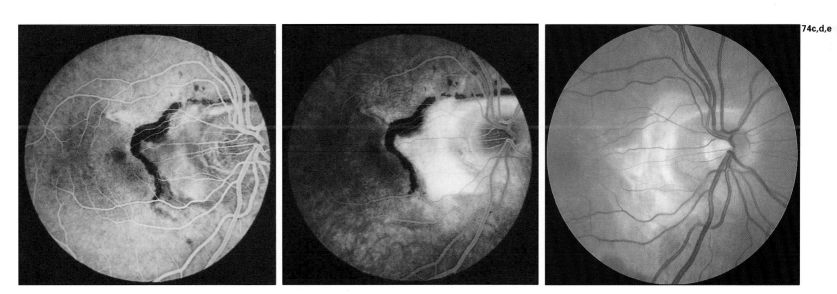

74 Peripapillary choroidal neovascularization. (**a**) A man of 30 presented with distortion and a visual acuity of 6/60. (**b,c,d**) There is an extensive peripapillary neovascular network with a border of haemorrhage. (**e**) The lesion became fibrotic, and eventually visual acuity improved to 6/9.

Central serous retinopathy

This condition (also known as central serous chorioretinopathy) affects people between the ages of 20 and 50, with a ratio of men to women of approximately 3:1. Symptoms include a partial central scotoma, distortion of central vision, micropsia, and an alteration in appreciation of colour. Fundus examination shows a smooth elevation of the retina at the macula which is best seen when viewed binocularly. The condition is self-limiting in the majority of cases, resolving within a few months leaving mild residual symptoms. Recurrences either in the same eye or in the fellow eye are not infrequent, and small patches of retinal pigment epithelial atrophy are often seen even when there have been no previous symptoms. Very occasionally, there may be a more chronic course with frequent recurrences or persistent symptoms where visual acuity remains permanently affected.

Fluorescein angiography shows a characteristic picture which is diagnostic. Typically there is one spot of hyperfluorescence which appears early then gradually enlarges as the dye fills the subretinal fluid-filled space (**75,76,77**). The boundary of the hyperfluorescent area appears 'fuzzy' and becomes less distinct with time. Eventually the entire fluid-filled area becomes hyperfluorescent, but it is not often necessary to wait more than two or three minutes after injection of the dye to recognize the evolving picture. Occasionally, a plume of hyperfluorescence is seen extending upwards from the original spot (**77**). This 'smoke stack' appearance is pathognomonic of the condition. In a few cases there may be more than one leaking point. Transmission defects at the site of pigment epithelial atrophy are common (**79**).

Some patients who present with similar symptoms are found on angiography to have small pigment epithelial detachments rather than classic central serous retinopathy 'hot spots'. Overlying serous detachment of the retina is often detected, and a central serous retinopathy spot demonstrated over the pigment epithelial detachment. The two lesions can coexist in the same eye, and as the clinical course and the profile of the patients affected is similar, they probably represent variations of the same disease (**78**).

In cases with definite symptoms and evidence of subretinal fluid but no detectable leakage on angiography, it can be assumed that the condition is no longer active, and resorption of subretinal fluid is to be anticipated.

Indications for angiography

A doubtful diagnosis Particular care should be taken in those patients at or above the upper limit of the age range usually affected. It can sometimes be difficult to distinguish the lesion clinically and angiographically from an early, small age-related neovascular network. Serial observation is then needed.

Treatment is being contemplated Although treatment with photocoagulation shortens the duration of an attack, long-term outcome and recurrence rates are unaffected. Treatment should be considered in patients where there appears to be no evidence of resolution after 4–6 months and where the symptoms interfere significantly with daily life. Only a few light laser burns are required. Fluorescein angiography is necessary to pinpoint the leaking spot.

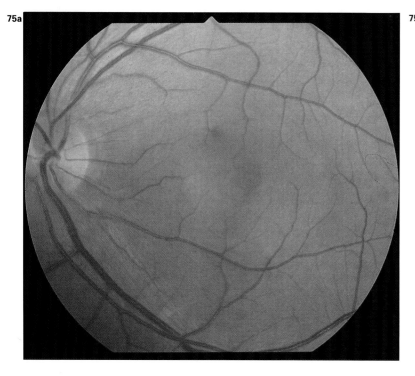

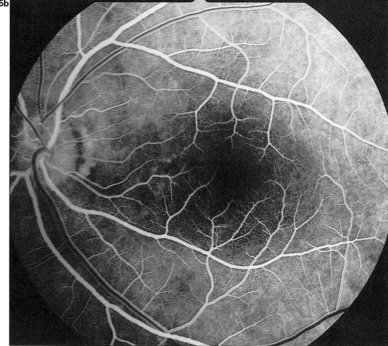

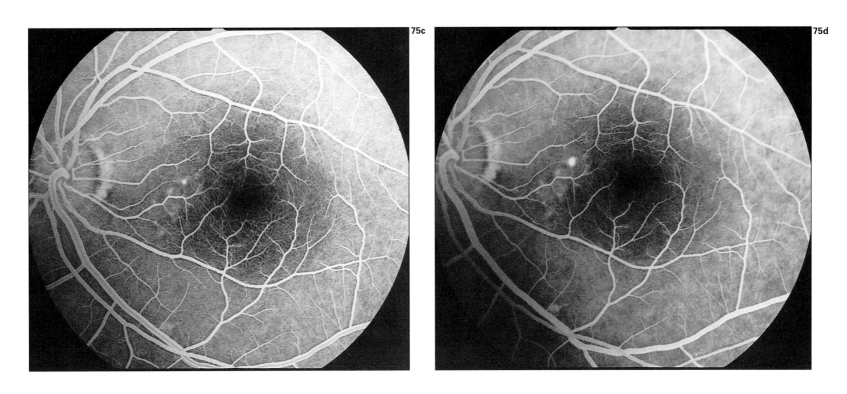

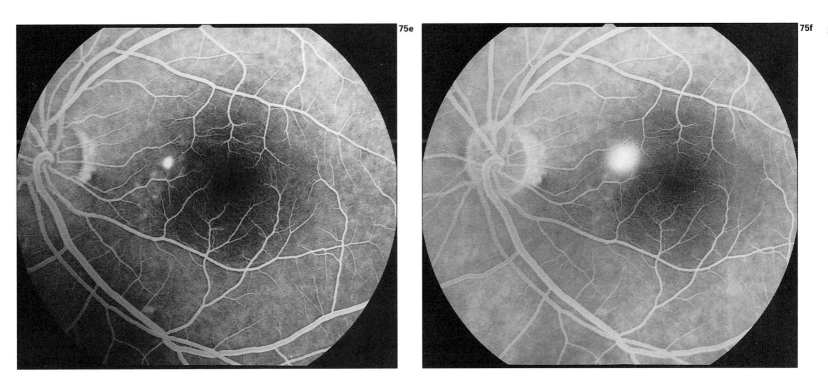

75 Central serous retinopathy. (**a**) A 43-year-old man noticed distortion, blurring and micropsia within an oval area in his central field of vision. Visual acuity was 6/12. As the symptoms had been present for over a year, angiography was performed with a view to laser treatment. (**b,c,d,e,f**) Sequential photographs show the appearance and gradual enlargement of a hyperfluorescent spot as dye diffuses into the subretinal fluid.

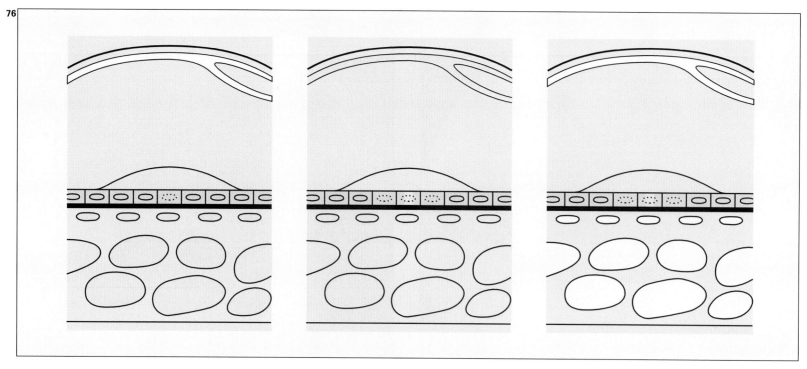

76 A diagram of central serous retinopathy to illustrate distribution of dye during the course of the angiogram.

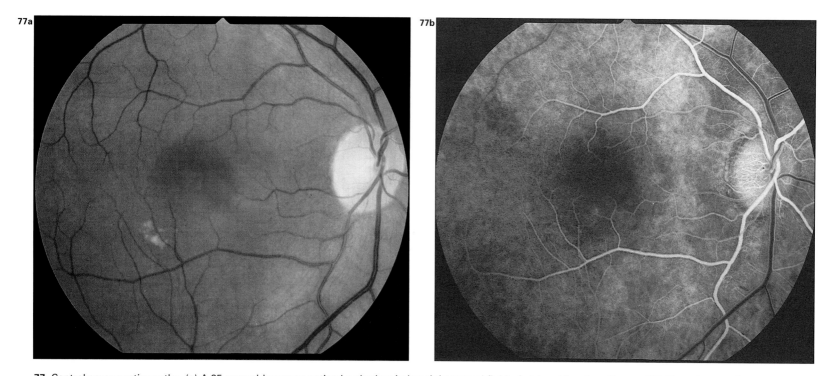

77 Central serous retinopathy. (**a**) A 35-year-old woman noticed a shadow in her right central field of vision. Visual acuity was 6/9. Over the next few months her symptoms disappeared and her visual acuity improved to 6/6. (**b,c,d,e,f**) In this case the spot did not enlarge concentrically but developed a vertical 'plume' or 'smoke stack', an appearance said to be pathognomonic of central serous retinopathy.

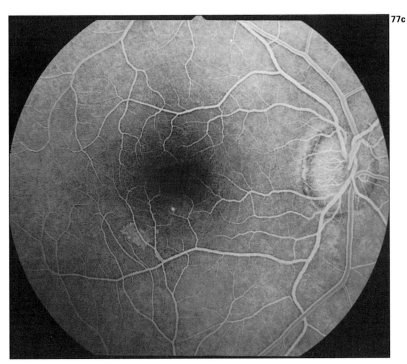

77c

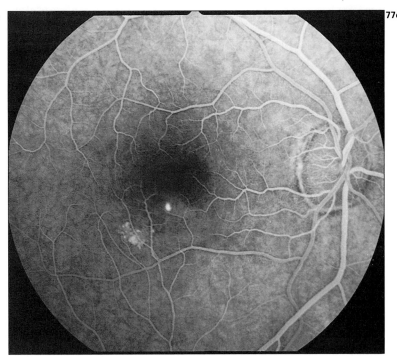

77d

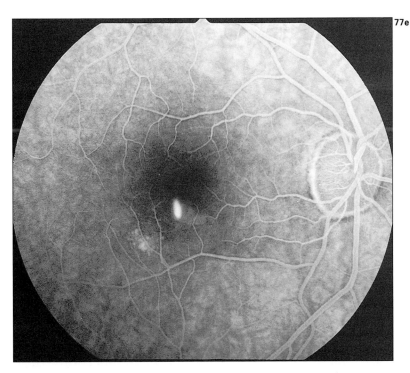

77e

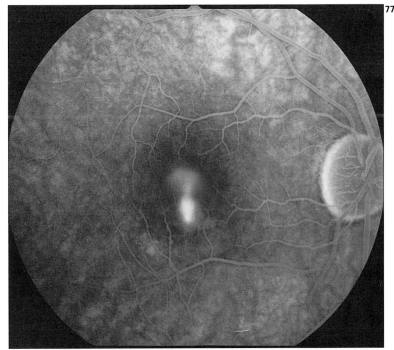

77f

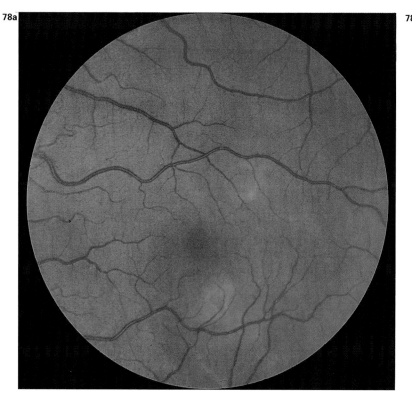

78a

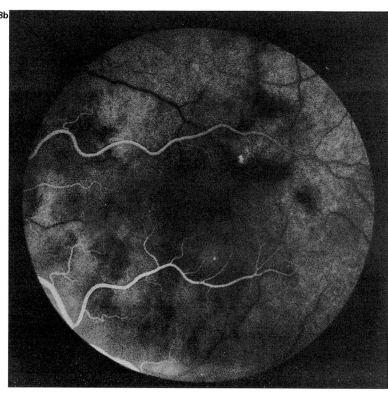

78b

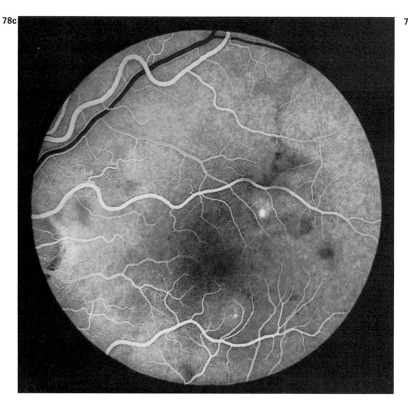

78c

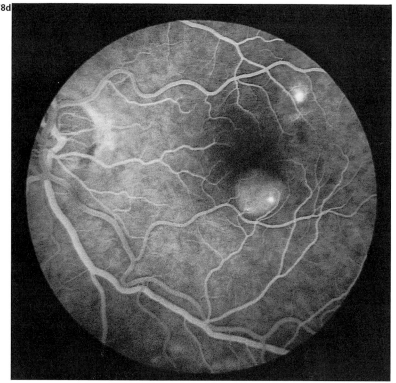

78d

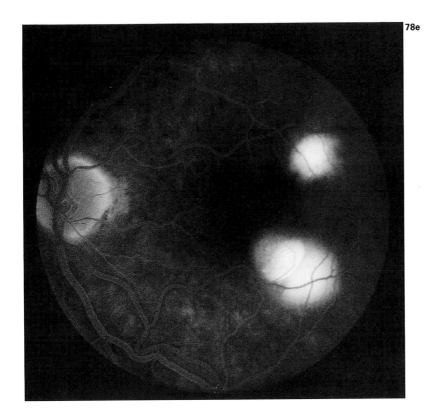

78 Central serous retinopathy/retinal pigment epithelial detachment. **(a)** A 40-year-old man noticed micropsia and dullness of colour. Visual acuity was 6/18. There was spontaneous improvement over the next few months and his visual acuity at discharge was 6/5. **(b,c,d,e)** In this case there are two separate lesions. In the lower one, the spot of leakage appears to overly a pigment epithelial detachment. The same probably also applies to the other one, although the margins of the pigment epithelial detachment are less easy to distinguish.

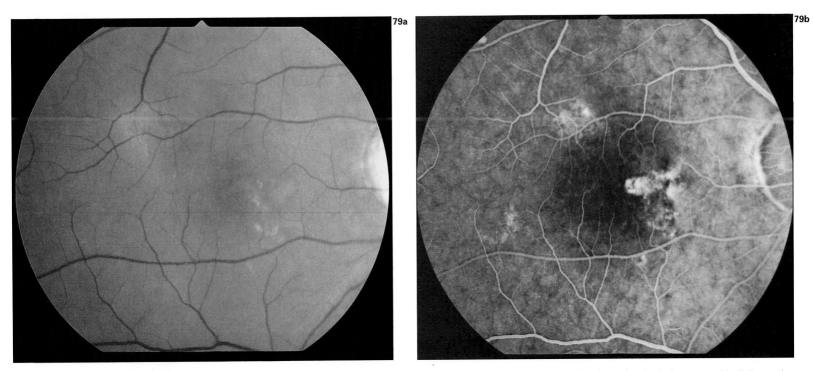

79 Resolved central serous retinopathy. This patient had suffered recurrent episodes of central serous retinopathy. Patches of retinal pigment epithelial atrophy remain and corresponding transmission defects are seen on the angiogram.

Macular holes

Idiopathic macular holes occur predominantly in women over the age of 60 years. Symptoms are rarely noticed in the early stages of evolution, particularly if one eye is affected. By the time the patient reports blurring and metamorphopsia, a full thickness hole is usually present. The hole is characteristically round, within the centre of the fovea, and surrounded by a ring of retinal detachment. It appears red in contrast to the greyish rim of retina and there are often yellow deposits within it at the level of the pigment epithelium. An overlying operculum is frequently seen.

Interest has recently focused on the stages of development of macular holes. A yellow spot or ring is first seen at the foveola with loss of the foveal depression (stage 1). Within a few weeks or months a hole starts to develop (stage 2), often at the edge of the ring, and enlarges until a round full-thickness lesion is present (stage 3). The presence of an operculum in front of the plane of the hole suggests local vitreous separation. However, in the majority of cases there is no separation of vitreous from the optic disc or the remaining macula. A few cases progress to posterior vitreous separation (stage 4). If the vitreous becomes detached from the fovea at the first stage of development without full-thickness hole formation, the lesion does not progress and the eye appears protected. It is suggested that macular holes result from changes in the prefoveal vitreous cortex, lead-ing to shrinkage. Anterior traction leads to foveal detachment, and tangential traction then causes hole formation.

The recognition of the importance of vitreoretinal traction as a cause of macular hole formation has led to advances in treatment. Vitrectomy has been used in the early stages of hole formation to prevent progression, and there is recent evidence that vitrectomy may improve visual acuity in cases with established holes by abolishing the rim of subretinal fluid.

Angiographic appearances

Angiography often shows no abnormal features in the first stage of hole formation, although sometimes there is faint central hyperfluorescence.

During stage 2, there is early hyperfluorescence in the area of the hole which fades during the course of the angiogram. An angiogram does not help to distinguish between the first and second stages.

Angiographic appearances corresponding to a full-thickness macular hole range from faint central hyperfluorescence to a more intense fluorescence associated with atrophic changes in the pigment epithelium and small, drusen-like deposits (80).

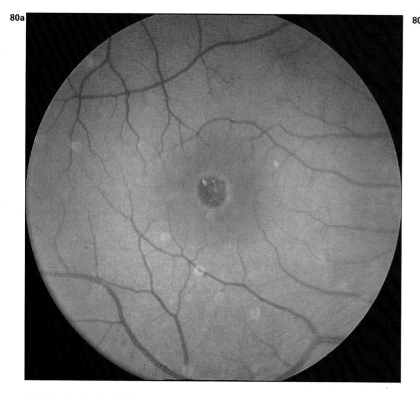

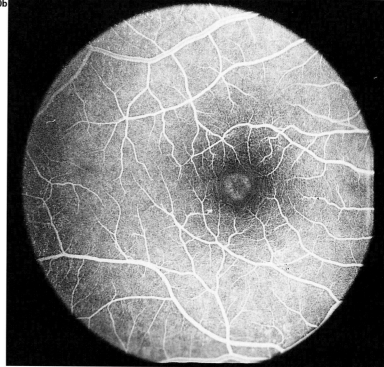

80 Macular hole. (**a**) A 72-year-old woman noticed blurring and distortion in her right eye on covering her left. Biomicroscopy demonstrated a full-thickness macular hole. (**b**) The area corresponding to the hole shows a patchy hyperfluorescence.

Epiretinal membranes

Many other terms have been used to describe this condition, including cellophane maculopathy, preretinal fibrosis, macular pucker and surface-wrinkling retinopathy. Cellular proliferation with membrane formation over the internal limiting membrane of the retina leads to wrinkling of the retina, with appearances at the macula ranging from a subtle alteration of the macular reflexes to marked distortion of the retinal vasculature with visible greyish membranes (**81,82,83**). In more severe cases, leakage from affected retinal vessels occurs (**82**), and contraction of the membrane sometimes leads to an appearance which mimics a macular hole (**83**). Several cell types have been implicated. Glial cells predominate in simple membranes, but in more severe cases fibroblasts, retinal pigment epithelial cells and macrophages have been detected.

Epiretinal membranes are idiopathic or secondary to other ocular disease, such as retinal vascular disease, retinal hole formation, following retinal detachment repair and ocular inflammatory disease. Symptoms most frequently described are distortion and blurring of vision. Idiopathic membranes are common in the elderly and in most cases are asymptomatic. In these cases there is a high incidence of coexisting posterior vitreous separation.

No treatment is usually required, but in the presence of significant symptoms such as distortion or a marked reduction in acuity, surgical removal or 'peeling' of the membrane is considered. Factors affecting outcome of surgery include membrane type, presence of cystoid macular oedema, pre-operative acuity and duration of symptoms.

Indications for angiography

Fluorescein angiography is useful in a number of circumstances in the investigation of symptomatic epiretinal membranes:

- To assess extent of retinal distortion.
- To determine presence and degree of vascular leakage.
- To distinguish between a pseudohole and a full-thickness macular hole.
- To investigate coexisting retinal vascular disease.

Angiographic appearance

The angiogram highlights the distorted retinal vessels and demonstrates straightening of surrounding vessels pulled centripetally. Capillary leakage, if present, is usually irregular and confined to the area of the pucker. A pseudohole does not reveal itself on angiography, whereas a full-thickness hole shows central hyperfluorescence as previously described.

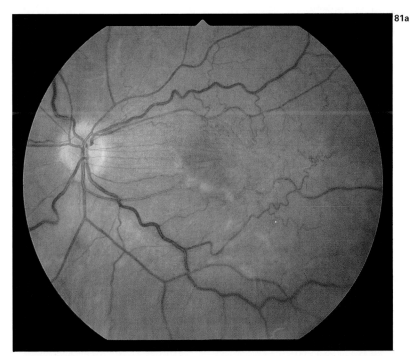
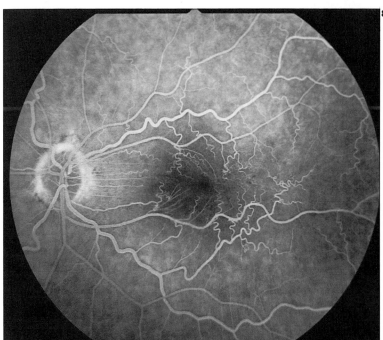

81 Epiretinal membrane. (**a**) A 64-year-old hypertensive woman complained of distortion. Her visual acuity was 6/12. (**b**) The angiogram emphasizes the dragging and straightening of the vessels arising from the disc and the increased tortuosity of the macular vessels.

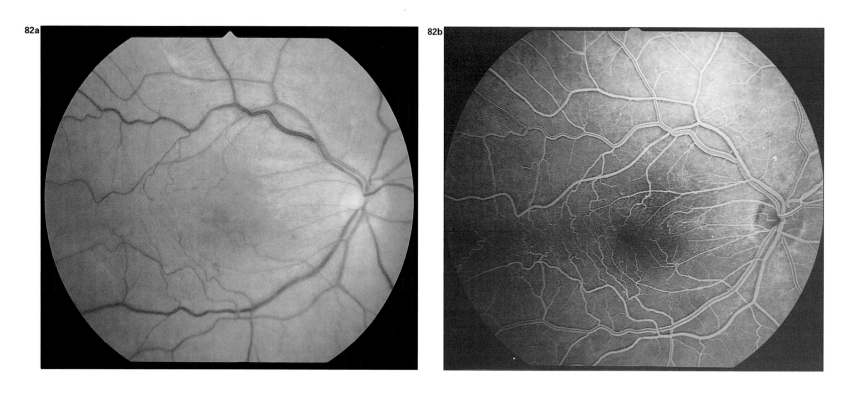

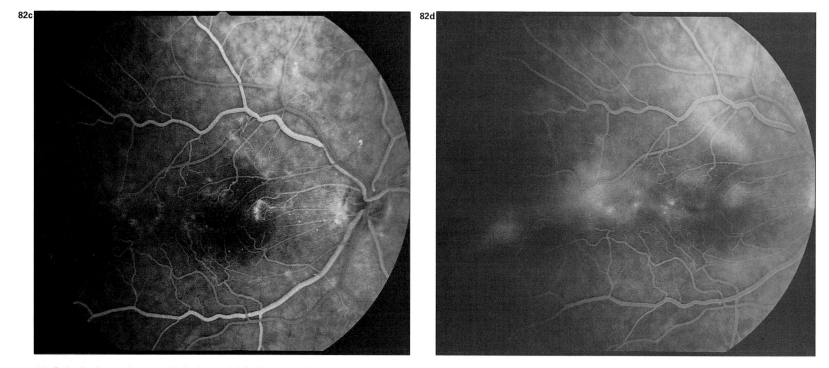

82 Epiretinal membrane with leakage. (**a**) A 70-year-old woman complained of blurred vision in her right eye. Visual acuity was 6/18. (**b,c,d**) In addition to the vascular distortion (see **81**), there is evidence of leakage.

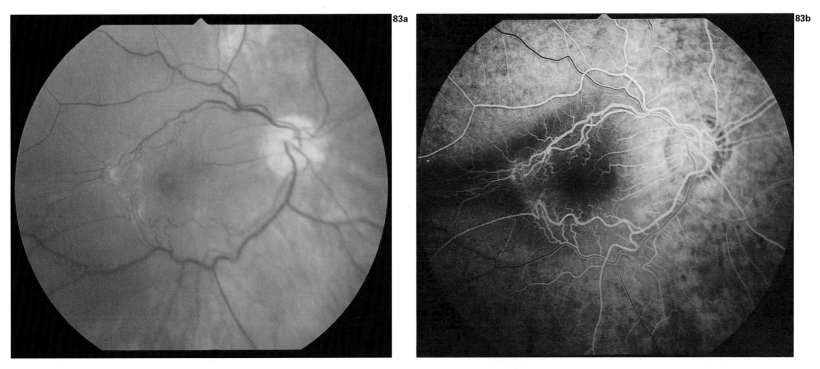

83 Epiretinal membrane with pseudohole. (a) A 45-year-old woman noticed a deterioration of vision with distortion. She was otherwise well and had no history of eye disease. Distortion of the retinal vasculature was noted, and the presence of a macular hole suspected, although her visual acuity remained at 6/9. (b) Angiography confirms the distortion of retinal vessels. The suspected hole does not appear on the angiogram and further careful clinical examination confirms that it is a pseudohole.

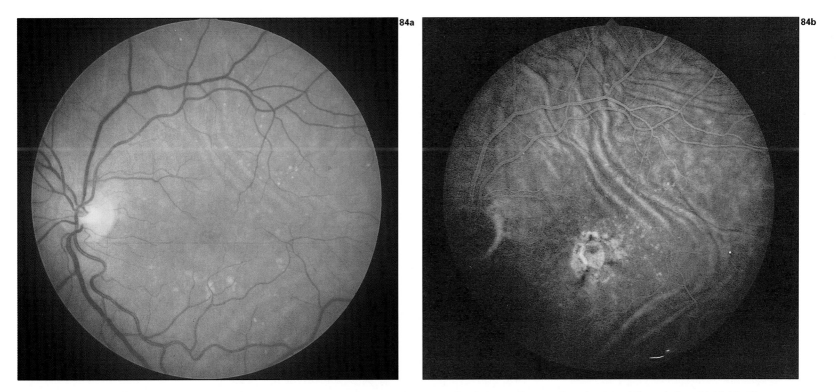

84 Choroidal folds. (a) A 73-year-old woman with unassociated atrophic age-related macular degeneration was found to have bilateral choroidal folds. There was no evidence of other ocular disease and an ultrasound test showed no evidence of a retro-orbital mass. She required a +3.50D lens to correct her hypermetropia. (b) Parallel light and dark lines correspond with peaks and troughs, respectively.

Chorioretinal folds

Folding of the choroid into parallel ridges may be either idiopathic, when it is often an incidental finding, or secondary to other ocular or orbital disease. Choroidal folds are found in association with orbital masses, thyroid eye disease, scleral inflammation, scleral explants, ocular hypotony, optic disc swelling, choroidal tumours and choroidal neovascularization. Hypermetropia frequently coexists in those cases where no underlying cause is evident.

Folds are linear or concentric to the optic disc. Angiography may demonstrate chorioretinal folds which are not obvious clinically and also help to distinguish between choroidal and retinal folds, as retinal folds are not visible on angiograms.

Angiographic appearances

The crests of the folds are hyperfluorescent because of the relative thinness of the pigment epithelium stretched over the fold. The troughs are hypofluorescent where the pigment epithelium is crowded, giving masking. The pattern of fluorescence remains constant, appearing and fading with the background choroidal fluorescence (**84**).

Bibliography

Bressler NM, Bressler SB, Gragoudas ES. Clinical characteristics of choroidal neovascular membranes. *Arch Ophthalmol* 1987;**105**:209–13.

Chisolm IH. The recurrence of neovascularization and late visual failure in senile disciform lesions. *Trans Ophthalmol Soc UK* 1983;**103**:354–9.

Chuang EL, Bird AC. The pathogenesis of tears of the retinal pigment epithelium. *Am J Ophthalmol* 1988;**105**:285–90.

Deutman AF, Kovacs B. Argon laser treatment in complications of angioid streaks. *Am J Ophthalmol* 1979;**88**:12–17.

Gass JDM. *Stereoscopic atlas of macular diseases*. St Louis: Mosby, 1987; Chapter 3 (Diseases causing choroidal exudative and haemorrhagic localised [disciform] detachment of the retina and pigment epithelium), Chapter 4 (Folds of the choroid and retina) and Chapter 12 (Macular dysfunction caused by vitreous and vitreoretinal interface abnormalities).

Gass JDM. Idiopathic senile macular hole: its early stages and pathogenesis. *Arch Ophthalmol* 1988;**106**:629–39.

Gelisken O, Hendrikse F, Deutman AF. A long-term follow-up study of laser coagulation of neovascular membranes in angioid streaks. *Am J Ophthalmol* 1988;**105**:299–303.

Grey RHB. Vascular disorders of the ocular fundus. London: Butterworths, 1991; Chapter 6 (The ageing macula and disciform degeneration).

Grey RHB, Bird AC, Chisolm IH. Senile disciform macular degeneration: features indicating suitability for photocoagulation. *Br J Ophthalmol* 1979;**63**:85–9.

Hilton GF. Late serosanguinous detachment of the macula after traumatic choroidal rupture. *Am J Ophthalmol* 1975;**79**:997–1000.

Kies JC, Bird AC. Juxtapapillary choroidal neovascularization in older patients. *Am J Ophthalmol* 1988;**105**:11–19.

Lopez PF, Green WR. Peripapillary subretinal neovascularization. A review. *Retina* 1992;**12**:147–71.

Macular Photocoagulation Study Group. The use of fundus photographs and fluorescein angiograms in the identification and treatment of choroidal neovascularization in the macular photocoagulation study. *Ophthalmology* 1989;**96**:1526–34.

Macular Photocoagulation Study Group. Krypton laser photocoagulation for neovascular lesions of age-related macular degeneration. *Arch Ophthalmol* 1990;**108**:816–24.

Maguire JI, Benson WE, Brown GC. Treatment of foveal pigment epithelial detachments with contiguous extrafoveal choroidal neovascular membranes. *Am J Ophthalmol* 1990;**109**:523–9.

Moorfields Macular Study Group. Treatment of senile disciform macular degeneration: a single-blind randomised trial by argon laser photocoagulation. *Br J Ophthalmol* 1982;**66**:745–53.

Moorfields Macular Study Group. Retinal pigment epithelial detachments in the elderly: a controlled trial of argon laser photocoagulation. *Br J Ophthalmol* 1982;**66**:1–16.

Pauleikhoff D, Chen JC, Chisolm IH, Bird AC. Choroidal perfusion abnormality with age-related Bruch's membrane change. *Am J Ophthalmol* 1990;**109**:211–17.

Robertson DH. Argon laser photocoagulation treatment in central serous chorioretinopathy. *Ophthalmology* 1986;**93**:972–4.

Ryan SJ. *Retina*. St Louis: Mosby, 1989; Chapter 64 (Age-related macular degeneration-atrophic form), Chapter 65 (Exudative age-related macular degeneration), Chapter 66 (Choroidal neovascular membrane in degenerative myopia), Chapter 67 (Central serous retinopathy), Chapter 68 (Macular hole), and Chapter 113 (Introduction to epiretinal membranes).

Shilling JS, Blach RK. Prognosis and therapy of angioid streaks. *Trans Ophthalmol Soc UK* 1975;**95**:310.

7 Inflammatory disorders

Angiography is important in the management of inflammatory fundus disorders and is used for diagnosis, determining disease activity and severity, and monitoring treatment. Appearances in some cases are specific and diagnostic, but certain manifestations of inflammation are common to a range of diseases.

This chapter begins with a summary of the nonspecific angiographic findings associated with many unrelated inflammatory disorders. This is followed by a more detailed description of different categories of ocular inflammatory disease, illustrating characteristic angiographic appearances.

Non-specific angiographic findings

Hyperpermeability of retinal vessels

Cystoid macular oedema and scattered foci of leakage from hyperpermeable capillaries over the posterior pole are a frequent finding in many inflammatory disorders, for example pars planitis, retinal vasculitis, and focal infections such as toxoplasmosis (see **89,97**).

Disc swelling

Swelling of the optic disc with dilatation and leakage of the disc capillaries is often part of the inflammatory process.

Retinal vasculitis

This is considered in greater detail under the heading of specific disorders, but it should be noted that retinal vasculitis may be part of virtually any severe intra-ocular inflammatory process.

Choroidal neovascularization

Choroidal neovascularization has been described as a complication of most inflammatory disorders, particularly those characterized by chorioretinal lesions leading to atrophy of the pigment epithelium at the macula (see **73**).

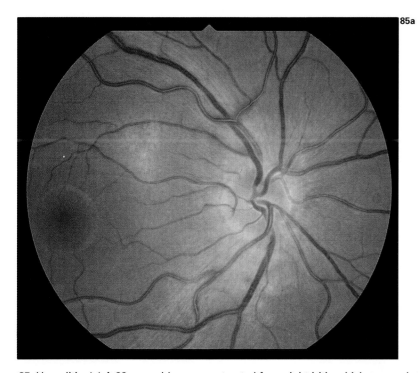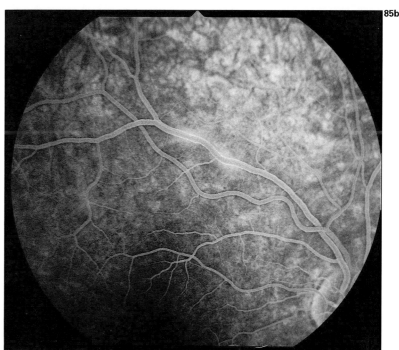

85 Vasculitis. (**a**) A 22-year-old man was treated for a right iritis which responded well to treatment. Soon after, the left eye became affected. Angiography was requested because disc swelling was suspected, but this was no longer apparent when the test was performed. There was no evidence of systemic disease and, to our knowledge, he has had no further symptoms three years later. (**b**) A late picture shows staining of the wall of a short segment of the upper temporal vein. There appears to be no other abnormality.

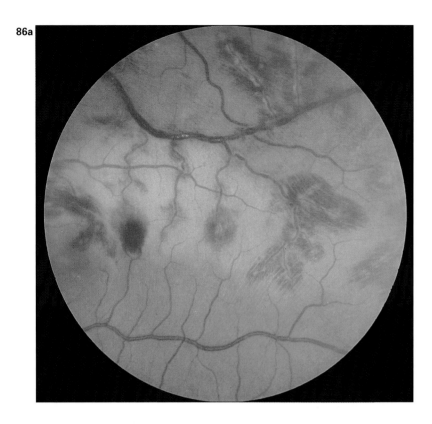

86a

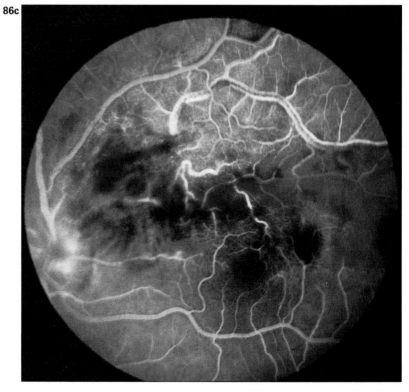

86 Vasculitis in Behçet's disease. (**a**) A 35-year-old woman had suffered from skin lesions and oral and perianal ulceration. She developed uveitis and an asymptomatic branch vein occlusion was discovered. A few months later, her vision fell to hand movements. (**b,c**) The pattern of haemorrhage suggests an occlusion of the upper temporal vein. The vein fills slowly and there is a large capillary filling defect. There is leakage from the disc. The vein and its tributaries demonstrate an intense and irregular hyperfluorescence.

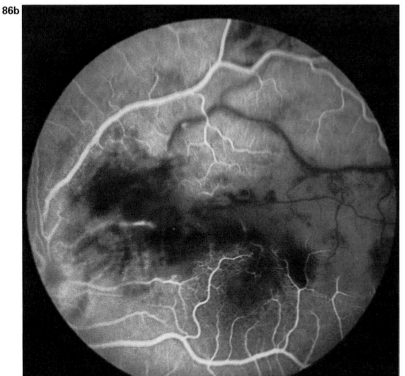

86b

86c

Examples of inflammatory disorders affecting the fundus

Retinal vasculitis

Retinal vasculitis occurs in many severe intra-ocular inflammatory processes (**85,86,87,88,89**). However, there is also a group of disorders, often with systemic manifestations, which are characterized by a vasculitic process, for example Behçet's disease (**86,87**), systemic lupus erythematosus, polyarteritis nodosa and sarcoidosis. Vasculitis is often accompanied by other signs of inflammation, such as uveitis or scleritis, but in other cases evidence of inflammation is restricted to a vitritis.

Vascular occlusive disease affecting the arterial or venous system is a common manifestation. Fundus examination shows haemorrhages, irregularities in the calibre of the larger vessels, sheathing, cotton wool spots and macular oedema. Retinal or disc neovascularization may develop with subsequent vitreous haemorrhage. Cells are present in the vitreous, and vitreous opacities may be dense enough to obscure fundus detail.

Fluorescein angiography demonstrates the nature and extent of retinal vascular involvement by detecting filling defects of the capillary bed and areas of hyperpermeability which are not obvious clinically (**85,86,87,88**). Unlike normal vessels, larger calibre vessels affected by a vasculitic process show hyperfluorescence of their walls with some spread beyond their margins, indicating uptake of dye and an increased permeability. These disturbances may be focal (**85**) or generalized. Angiography can often detect cystoid macular oedema or areas of retinal or choroidal neovascularization where vitreous opacities or haemorrhage obscure the fundus.

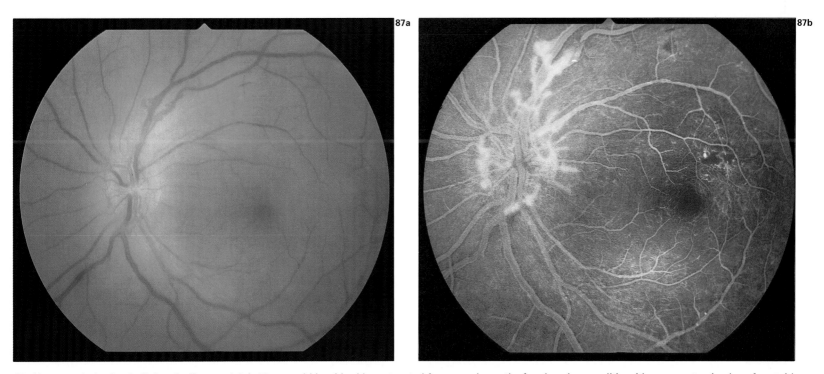

87 Neovascularization in Behçet's disease. (**a**) A 42-year-old Iraqi had been treated for several months for chronic vasculitis with recurrent episodes of cystoid macular oedema. His ocular symptoms responded to treatment with cyclosporin and systemic steroids. Other symptoms included skin rashes and joint pains. (**b**) The larger vessels show irregularity of calibre. The capillary bed around the fovea, particularly on the temporal side, is abnormal with a well-defined small filling defect. There is neovascularization at the disc.

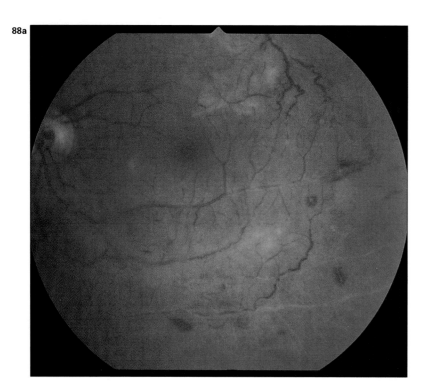

Eales' disease

Eales' disease affects young adults and is more common in India and the Middle East. Patients present most frequently with recurrent vitreous haemorrhages and are found to have extensive peripheral retinal non-perfusion, vascular sheathing and neovascularization (**88**). Signs of intermittent ocular inflammation, including uveitis, vitritis and cystoid macular oedema, are common in the early stages of the disease but often absent at the time of presentation. The cause is unknown and the diagnosis is made after exclusion of other conditions associated with retinal vasculitis and neovascularization. An association with tuberculosis is described but the nature of the relationship is not clear.

Infections

A large variety of organisms produce infective retinitis and chorioretinitis, including bacteria, viruses, rickettsial organisms, and parasites.

The most common infecting organism is the protozoan *Toxoplasma gondii*. The infection is usually acquired *in utero*, and lies dormant for many years. White fluffy areas of acute retinitis occur, often at the edge of an old chorioretinal scar. There are associated cells in the vitreous and, in cases of severe inflammation, there may be cystoid macular oedema (**89**).

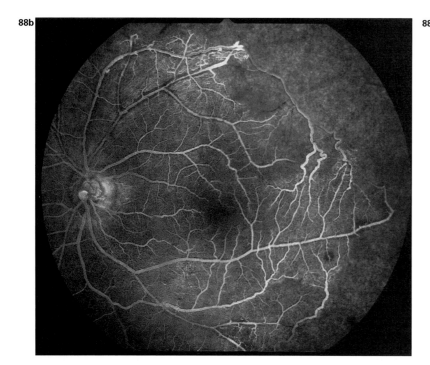

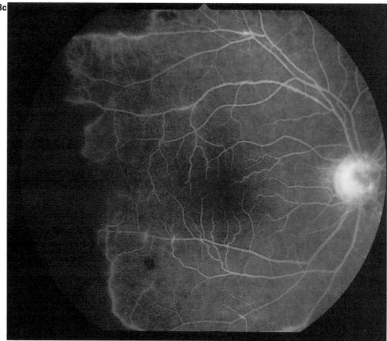

88 Retinal vasculitis in suspected Eales' disease. (**a**) A 40-year-old man, a visitor from the Middle East, had suffered from intermittent blurring of vision over the past few months. Intensive investigation revealed no evidence of any systemic disorder. (**b**) Angiography emphasizes the irregularity in calibre of the larger retinal vessels. There is total absence of filling of retinal vessels in the periphery. (**c**) A later picture of the right eye demonstrates clearly the boundary between perfused and nonperfused retinal vasculature. There is staining of vessel walls, particularly near the ischaemic areas. Intense hyperfluorescence at the disc suggests leakage of dye.

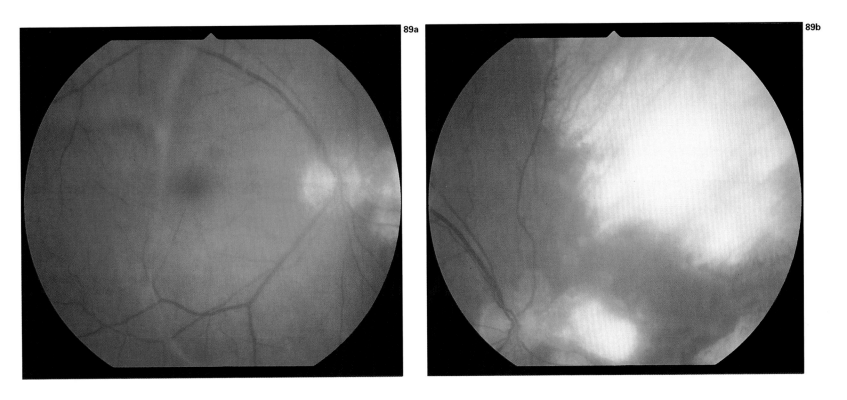

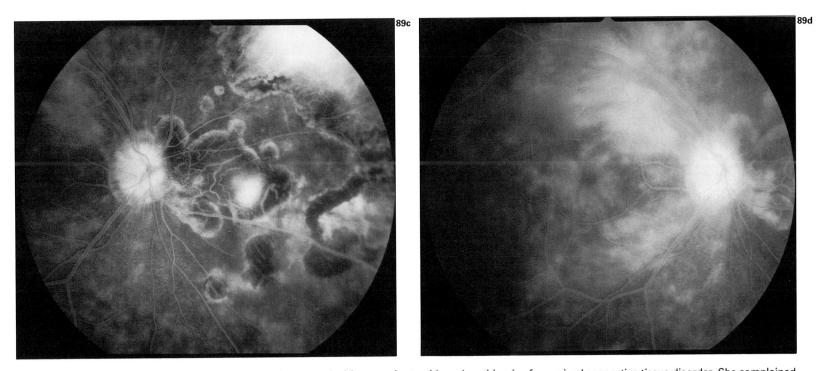

89 Toxoplasmosis. (**a,b**) A 42-year-old woman was being treated with systemic steroids and azathioprine for a mixed connective tissue disorder. She complained of deterioration of vision in her right eye. Her left fundus was quite normal. On the right there were a number of fluffy white lesions adjacent to areas of chorioretinal scarring. The appearances clinically were those of toxoplasmosis and it was assumed that the severity of the recurrence was related to the immunosuppressive therapy she was using. (**c**) The active chorioretinal lesions are highly fluorescent. Choroidal vessels can be seen at the base of the long-standing chorioretinal scar just nasal to the disc. (**d**) There is intense hyperfluorescence of the disc, cystoid macular oedema, and evidence of fluorescein leakage from the retinal vasculature scattered over the posterior pole.

Opportunistic ocular infections have become more common with the spread of the human immunodeficiency virus (HIV). A high proportion of patients with the acquired immune deficiency syndrome (AIDS) develop a retinopathy which has not as yet been attributed to secondary infection (**90**). Cotton wool spots and haemorrhage are frequent findings and angiography demonstrates microvascular abnormalities such as microaneurysms, telangiectasia and small areas of capillary loss similar to those seen in diabetes. This form of retinopathy does not appear to progress or produce visual symptoms.

The most important cause of infectious retinopathy in AIDS is the cytomegalovirus (CMV). CMV gives rise to a necrotizing retinitis which is responsible for severe visual loss and is often the presenting feature of generalized CMV disease (**91**). Fundus examination shows white areas associated with retinal haemorrhages and vascular sheathing. Complications include exudative and rhegmatogenous retinal detachments. Fluorescein angiography demonstrates retinal vascular filling defects and leakage, and is useful in those early cases where the lesions are confined to the peripheral retina.

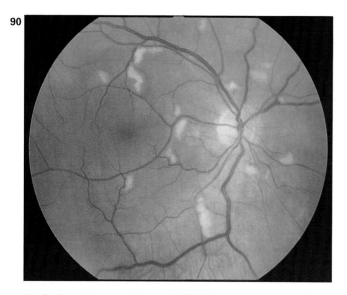

90 Retinopathy associated with HIV infection. Cotton wool spots in a patient known to be HIV positive. (Courtesy of Dr S Glover.)

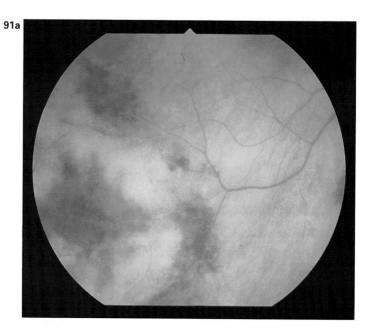

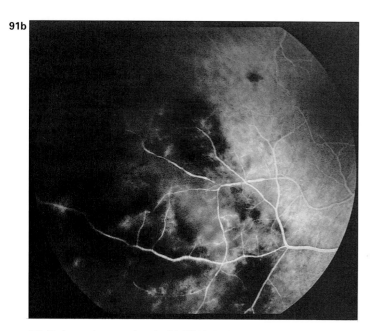

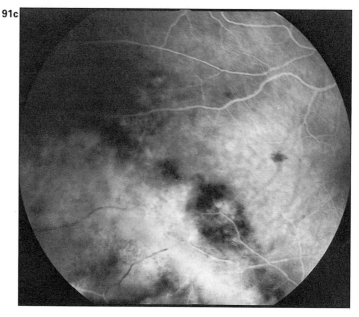

91 Retinopathy associated with HIV infection. (**a**) Cytomegalovirus infection in a patient with AIDS. (**b**) Angiogram corresponding with area of retinitis illustrated in (**a**). Retinal vessels show irregularities of fluorescence and calibre as they pass through the affected area. The more peripheral branches fail to fill. Hypofluorescence corresponds with areas of retinal haemorrhage and with retinal vascular filling defects. (**c**) Occluded vessels show up against a background of hyperfluorescence at three minutes. (Courtesy of Dr S Glover.)

The choroid in inflammatory disorders

The choroid is primarily affected by infection with a number of organisms, including bacteria, yeasts, fungi and parasites, although many of these infections are rare in the developed world. It is almost always involved in infections primarily affecting the neuroretina (see above) and is important in the pathogenesis of the disorders affecting the retinal pigment epithelium (discussed below).

The angiographic appearance of choroidal granulomas in sarcoid disease is shown below (**92**). Choroidal granulomas occur in only 5% of cases of ocular sarcoid. Retinal vasculitis and optic neuropathy are more common manifestations (**93**).

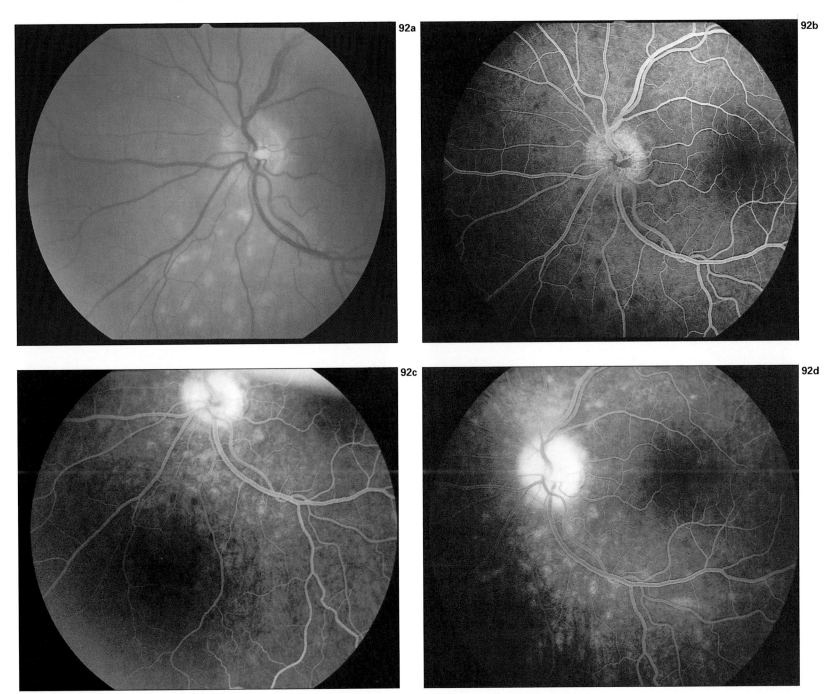

92 Sarcoid disease – choroidal granulomas. (**a**) A 34-year-old man presented with a low grade bilateral uveitis. Fundus examination showed scattered choroidal granulomas. Lung markings were abnormally pronounced on chest X-ray and angiotensin-converting enzyme levels were high. (**b**) The prepapillary capillaries are dilated. Many hypofluorescent patches are seen which persist. (**c,d**) The disc is intensely fluorescent as dye leaks from dilated capillaries. Scattered small hyperfluorescent patches appear during the transit and persist in the late frames.

Disorders of the choroid and retinal pigment epithelium

Harada's disease

Harada's disease affects predominantly black and oriental races. Unilateral or bilateral serous retinal detachments, often accompanied by vitritis and disc swelling, lead to rapid and profound loss of vision. Symptoms suggesting central nervous system involvement, such as headache and vomiting, are often present. Some patients develop severe anterior uveitis, poliosis, vitiligo and hyperacusis which, together with the signs of Harada's disease, constitute the Vogt–Koyanagi syndrome.

Grey or pale yellow elevations at the level of the pigment epithelium are associated with overlying detachment of the neuroretina. Large bullous detachments of the retina may develop. Fluorescein angiography shows patchy filling of the choroid. During the course of the angiogram, small spots of hyperfluorescence and larger irregular areas of hyperfluorescence develop (94). In late pictures, dye may be seen in the subretinal exudate. Leakage from the disc is often present.

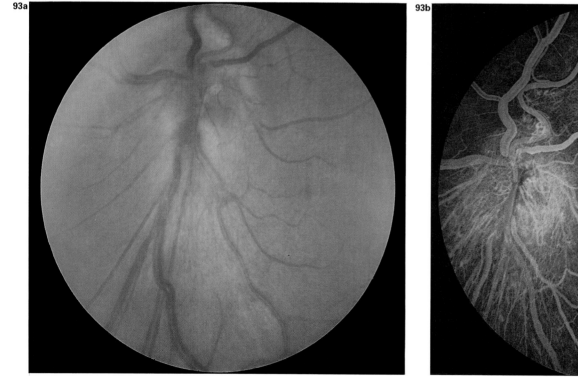
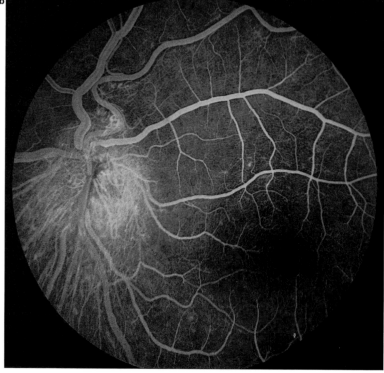

93 Sarcoid disease – optic neuropathy. (**a**) A woman with known sarcoid disease presented with uveitis and optic disc swelling. There was evidence of vasculitis in the peripheral retina. (**b**) The disc shows asymmetric swelling. Overlying vessels are dilated. Sarcoid infiltration of the optic nerve was suspected.

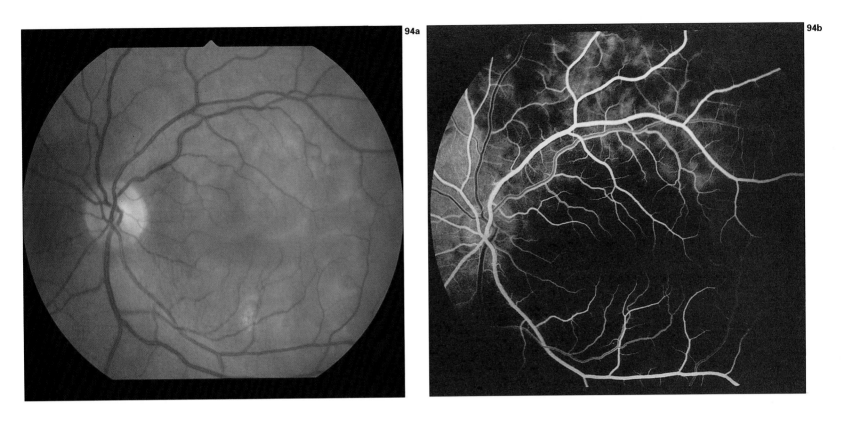

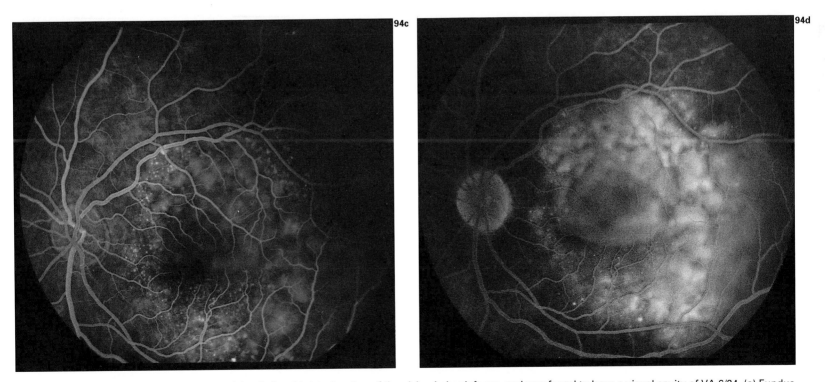

94 Harada's disease. A young woman complained of rapid deterioration of the vision in her left eye, and was found to have a visual acuity of VA 6/24. (**a**) Fundus examination showed areas of pallor and a serous detachment of the retina. (**b,c,d**) Although the angiographic appearances were typical of Harada's disease, she was otherwise completely asymptomatic and made a full recovery within six weeks, and without treatment.

Acute posterior multifocal placoid pigment epitheliopathy

Acute posterior multifocal placoid pigment epitheliopathy (APMPPE) affects young adults of both sexes. A flu-like illness may precede the condition, and there have been some reports of an accompanying meningitis or meningoencephelitis. The cause is unknown. Visual symptoms at the onset are variable, but visual acuity can drop to single figures in the worse affected eye if the fovea is involved. In the early stages the fundus shows white/cream patches at the posterior pole, ⅛–¼ disc diameters in width, which tend to become confluent. Over the following weeks there is resolution of symptoms, and visual acuity returns to normal or near normal levels in most cases. Fundus abnormalities in the form of pigment epithelial atrophy and pigment clumping sometimes remain, but often clear completely. The atrophy is more obvious on angiography than on ophthalmoscopy.

Angiographic appearances The pale lesions of APMPPE are initially hypofluorescent, but become hyperfluorescent during the course of the angiogram and remain fluorescent in the late frames (**95**). The reason for these angiographic appearances remains uncertain. One suggestion has been that the primary lesion is within the pigment epithelium and that the hypofluorescence is due to masking by the swollen cells which later stain with absorbed dye. An alternative view, for which there is increasing evidence, is that small filling defects of the choriocapillaris lobules give rise to the hypofluorescent spots. The overlying pigment epithelium is infarcted with late hyperfluorescence caused by staining of the damaged cells.

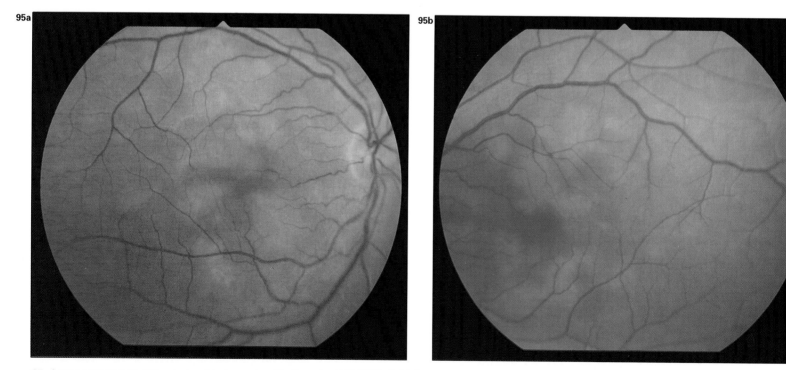

95 Acute posterior multifocal placoid pigment epitheliopathy (APMPPE). (**a,b**) A man of 28 noticed a rapid deterioration of vision in his right eye a week after a minor upper respiratory tract infection. Visual acuity was 6/36, 6/12. Over the next two months the right acuity improved to 6/12.

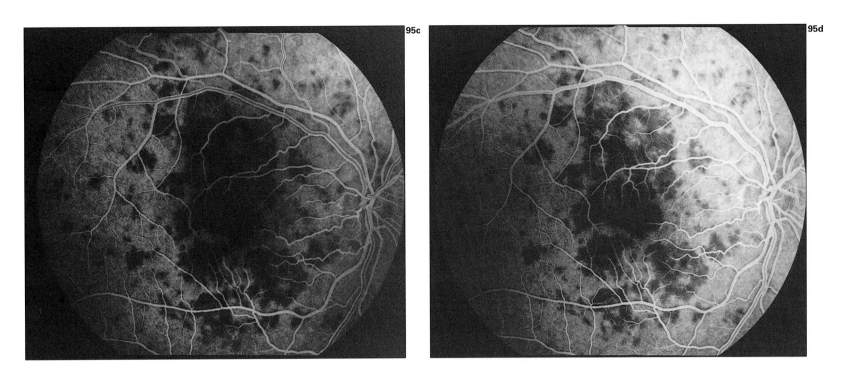

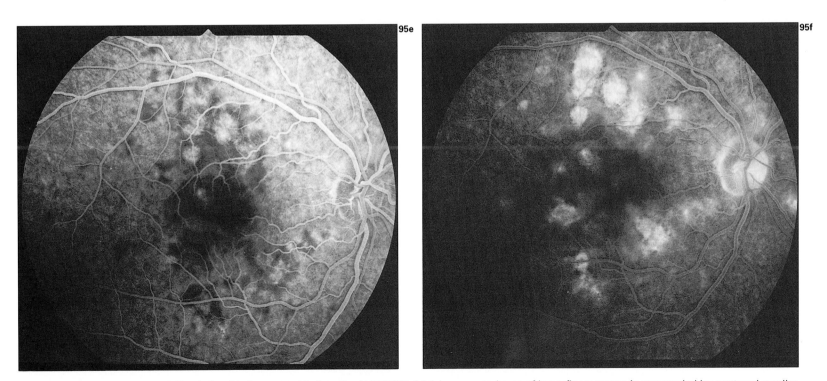

95 (contd) Acute posterior multifocal placoid pigment epitheliopathy (APMPPE). (**c**) A large central area of hyperfluorescence is surrounded by scattered smaller lesions. (**d**) The hypofluorescent areas are more sharply demarcated against the increasing background fluorescence. (**e**) Patches of fluorescence are developing within the previously hypofluorescent areas. (**f**) At four minutes there has been further increase in hyperfluorescence at the site of previously dark areas, although the sizes and shapes of the hyperfluorescent patches do not exactly match those of the original lesions.

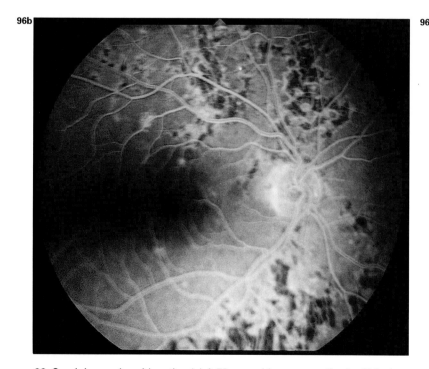

Serpiginous choroiditis (geographic choroidopathy)

Serpiginous choroiditis is a chronic inflammatory condition affecting the choroid and pigment epithelium in adults. The acute lesion – a pale area at the level of the pigment epithelium – resolves leaving a chorioretinal scar. Over a period of months or years further lesions arise, often adjacent to areas of previous scarring giving rise to a geographic or serpiginous pattern. Vision is affected if the fovea is involved. The condition is bilateral, but it is unusual for central vision to be affected in both eyes. Vitritis is relatively common, and retinal vasculitis has been described. Subsequent choroidal neovascularization is an important cause of visual loss.

The acute lesions are hypofluorescent in the early transit but later stain with dye. The older, atrophic areas show evidence of destruction of the choroid. They are hypofluorescent in the early stages of the angiogram, but later show staining extending from the margins inwards (96). Fluorescein angiography is particularly useful in determining whether loss of vision is due to progression of the underlying disease or to the development of choroidal neovascularization.

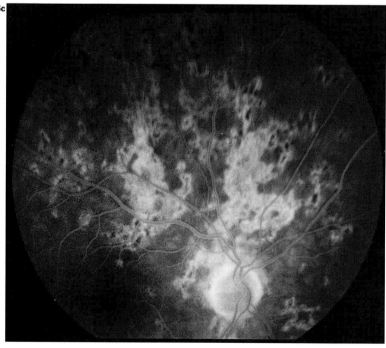

96 Serpiginous choroidopathy. **(a)** A 52-year-old woman noticed a flickering sensation in her right eye. Visual acuity was 6/6, 6/6. A pattern of irregular atrophy radiated from both discs. The maculae were not involved. **(b)** No active lesion is demonstrated in this case. The geographic lesions are hypofluorescent and choroidal vessels can be seen denoting destruction of the choriocapillaris and pigment epithelium. Satellite or skip lesions are present. **(c)** Staining of fibrous tissue leads to hyperfluorescence around and within lesions.

Birdshot chorioretinopathy

Birdshot chorioretinopathy is a rare disorder, characterized by the presence of pale yellow patches of depigmentation at the level of the choroid. Signs of inflammation include vitritis, disc swelling and cystoid macular oedema. Choroidal neovascularization may develop. The cause is unknown, but there is a strong association with the tissue type HLA–A29.

Angiography sometimes shows areas of hypofluorescence corresponding to the pale areas which become slightly hyperfluorescent in the late pictures. However, often there is no angiographic abnormality at the site of the patches. Angiographic features indicating disc oedema and cystoid macular oedema are often present (**97**).

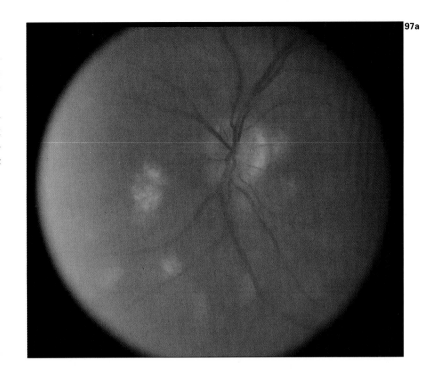

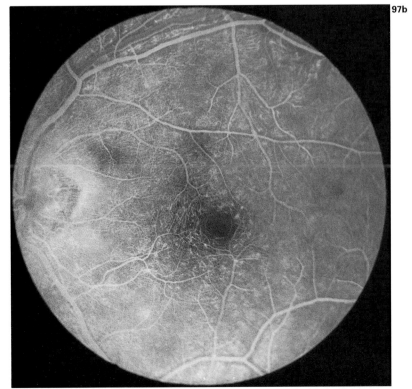

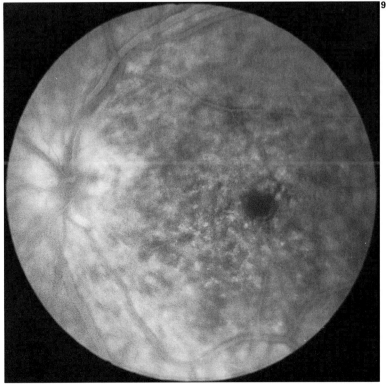

97 Birdshot chorioretinopathy. (**a**) A 72-year-old man noticed a gradual deterioration of vision associated with floaters. Visual acuity was 6/60, 6/60. The eyes appeared white, but vitreous cells and opacities were present. The pale yellow lesions radiated from the disc into the mid-periphery. The right eye showed a similar appearance to the left. (**b,c**) There is leakage from the disc and retinal vasculature. The typical petaloid pattern developed in later frames (not included). There are no angiographic features which correspond to the pale fundus lesions in this case.

Bibliography

Gass JDM. A fluorescein angiographic study of macular dysfunction secondary to retinal vascular disease. VI. X-ray irradiation, carotid artery occlusion, collagen vascular disease, and vitritis. *Arch Ophthalmol* 1968; **80**:606–17.

Gass JDM. *Stereoscopic atlas of macular diseases*. St Louis: Mosby, 1987; Chapter 3 (Diseases causing choroidal exudative and hemorrhagic localised [disciform] detachment of the retina and pigment epithelium) and Chapter 7 (Inflammatory diseases of the retina and choroid).

Gold DH, Weingeist TA. *The eye in systemic disease*. Philadelphia: JB Lippincott, 1990; Chapter 26 (Systemic lupus erythematosus), Chapter 92 (Behçet's syndrome) and Chapter 96 (Sarcoidosis).

Grey RHB. *Vascular disorders of the ocular fundus*. London: Butterworths, 1991; Chapter 8 (Retinal vasculitis and related disorders).

Jabs DA, Johns CJ. Ocular involvement in chronic sarcoidosis. *Am J Ophthalmol* 1986; **102**:302–7.

Rubsamen PE, Gass JDM. Vogt–Koyanagi–Harada Syndrome. Clinical course, therapy, and long-term visual outcome. *Arch Ophthalmol* 1991; **109**:682–7.

Ryan SJ. *Retina*. St Louis: Mosby, 1989; Chapter 79 (The Rheumatic Diseases) and Section 6 (Inflammatory disease).

Sanders MD, Shilling JS. Retinal, choroidal and optic disc involvement in sarcoidosis. *Trans Ophthalmol Soc UK* 1976; **96**:140.

Wolf MD, Alward WLM, Folk JC. Long-term visual function in acute posterior multifocal placoid pigment epitheliopathy. *Arch Ophthalmol* 1991; **109**:800–803.

Young NJA, Bird AC, Sehmi K. Pigment epithelial diseases with abnormal choroidal perfusion. *Am J Ophthalmol* 1980; **90**:607–18.

8 Retinal dystrophies

The diagnosis of retinal dystrophies is based on the fundus appearance, family history and patterns of visual and electrophysiological dysfunction. Occasionally, however, angiography demonstrates abnormalities before they are apparent on fundoscopy, or reveals changes that are more widespread than suspected. It is outside the scope of this book to discuss in detail the full diversity of the conditions included under this heading. We have therefore restricted the text to those most commonly seen.

Cone dystrophy/bull's eye maculopathy

This group of inherited dystrophies is characterized by evidence of involvement of the cone system, including symptoms of central or paracentral scotoma, defects in colour vision, and abnormal electroretinography. These dystrophies are dominantly or recessively inherited and are often sporadic. A variety of fundus changes are described, but a common early sign is a ring of parafoveal pigment epithelial atrophy, termed Bull's eye maculopathy. In the early stages, fundus changes are often subtle (**98**). Later, full thickness retinal pigment epithelial atrophy at the macula often develops.

Fluorescein angiography is helpful in detecting a maculopathy before it is obvious ophthalmoscopically. In some families a silent choroid is detected.

Stargardt's disease and fundus flavimaculatus

Stargardt's disease is an autosomally recessive, inherited macular degeneration associated with pale flecks at the level of the pigment epithelium (**99**). Fundus flavimaculatus describes the appearance of the yellow-flecked fundus. Although these terms are often used interchangeably, flecks can exist without atrophy at the macula, and it is not certain that such flecks form part of the same disease process. However, many people who present with fundus flavimaculatus alone do ultimately develop macular degeneration.

In Stargardt's disease, gradual deterioration of vision occurs during childhood or early adulthood, and can predate any ophthalmoscopic signs. At this stage, angiography may be helpful in confirming atrophy of the retinal pigment epithelium. Later, atrophy becomes apparent on ophthalmoscopy, with surrounding yellow flecks which may extend to involve the mid-periphery. The flecks are hypofluorescent or hyperfluorescent. When hyperfluorescent, the outline is irregular and does not correspond exactly with the visible lesions, thus distinguishing them from drusen.

In some cases, choroidal fluorescence is obscured in the peripheral part of the macula. This sign is known as the 'dark' or 'silent' choroid and is thought to be caused by deposition of lipofuscin within retinal pigment epithelial cells, giving rise to masking.

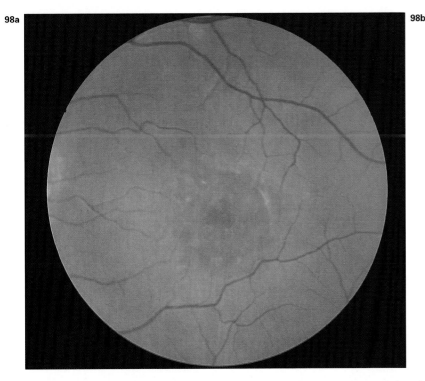

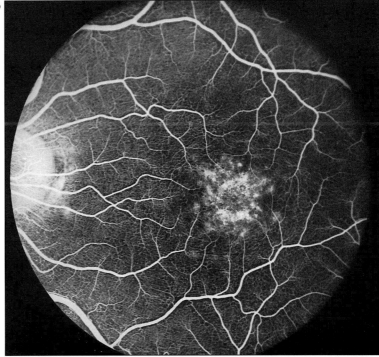

98 Cone dystrophy. (**a**) An 18-year-old girl complained of deteriorating central acuity and colour vision. Her symptoms were most pronounced in bright illumination. Visual acuity was 6/18, 6/18. Two sisters were similarly affected. (**b**) The pattern of atrophy is more striking on angiography than on ophthalmoscopic examination and colour photography. Background fluorescence is reduced. The changes were symmetrical in the two eyes.

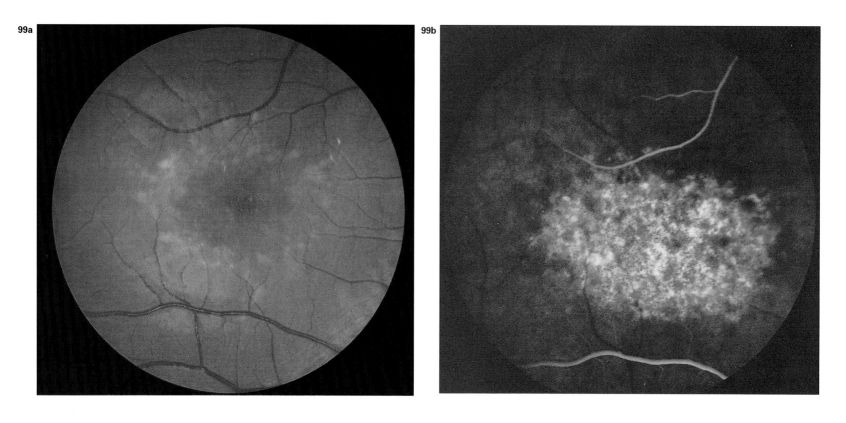

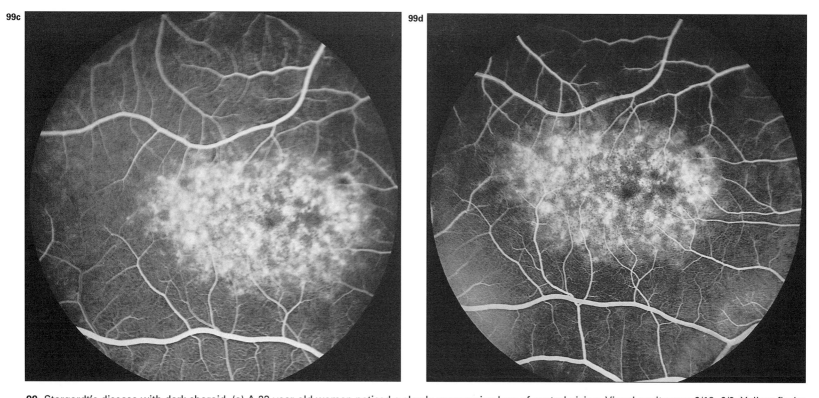

99 Stargardt's disease with dark choroid. (**a**) A 23-year-old woman noticed a slowly progressive loss of central vision. Visual acuity was 6/18, 6/9. Yellow flecks surround the atrophic macular lesion, although they do not extend into the periphery in this case. (**b,c,d**) There is a characteristically shaped patch of atrophic change at the macula. The patchy hyperfluorescence does not correspond with the yellow flecks. The surrounding picture appears dark and the retinal capillaries are more prominent. This is an example of the 'dark' or 'silent' choroid sign where the pigment epithelium blocks underlying choroidal fluorescence.

Best's disease (vitelliform macular dystrophy)

Best's disease is dominantly inherited, but penetrance of the gene is variable. During the first decade, a well-circumscribed round or oval yellowish lesion appears at the macula. At this stage the visual acuity is usually normal. In time, the smooth yellow dome becomes irregular, sometimes passing through a pseudohypopyon stage in which yellow material collects inferiorly, forming a fluid level. Eventually an oval area of pigment epithelial atrophy or fibrosis secondary to choroidal neovascularization remains. Although central visual acuity sometimes drops to 6/60 or less, vision is often better than this in at least one eye (**100,101**).

The diagnosis is apparent from the clinical appearance and family history. A subnormal electro-oculogram in the presence of a normal electroretinogram confirms the diagnosis. Carriers of the abnormal gene have an abnormal electro-oculogram in the absence of fundus changes.

Angiographic appearances

At the vitelliform stage, when the lesion has the appearance of a yellow disc, it is hypofluorescent on angiography with masking of choroidal hyperfluorescence (**100**). As the vitelliform lesion becomes disrupted, there is hyperfluorescence associated with pigment epithelial atrophy. During progression of the lesion, typical changes of choroidal neovascularization are sometimes demonstrated, and occult neovascularization is often suspected. Well defined hyperfluorescence develops later, associated with transmission defects in the pigment epithelium and staining of subretinal fibrous tissue.

100a

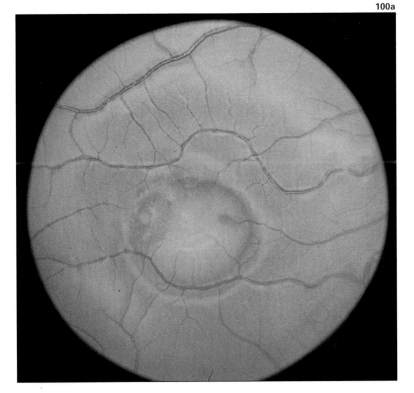

100b

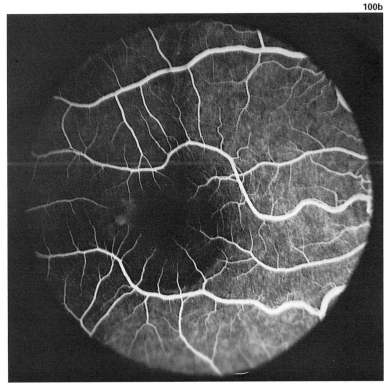

100 Best's disease: vitelliform stage. (**a**) A typical vitelliform lesion. (**b**) Apart from slight hypofluorescence due to masking, there is no angiographic abnormality.

Adult onset foveomacular vitelliform dystrophy

This condition presents in adulthood with a mild to moderate deterioration of vision. Pale circular macular lesions are seen which are smaller than those present at the vitelliform stage of Best's disease (**102**). They may be single or multiple, uniocular or binocular. Electro-oculograms are normal or reduced.

Retinitis pigmentosa

The term retinitis pigmentosa is used to describe a wide range of retinal dystrophies with different clinical features and modes of inheritance.

Angiography is not required for diagnosis, which is made on the basis of fundus appearance, visual function, electrodiagnostic tests and family history. However, angiography is useful in the detection and the assessment of severity of associated capillary permeability and cystoid macular oedema. These changes are more common than previously suspected. In some cases acetazolamide has been shown to be of value in the treatment of this complication, and angiography has a role in monitoring the response.

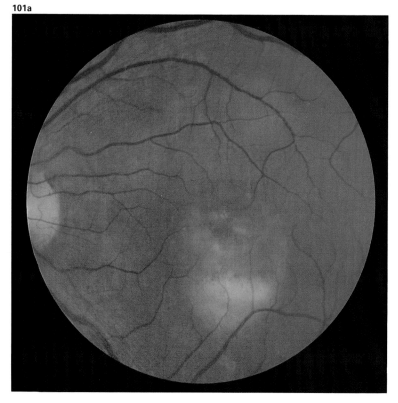

101a

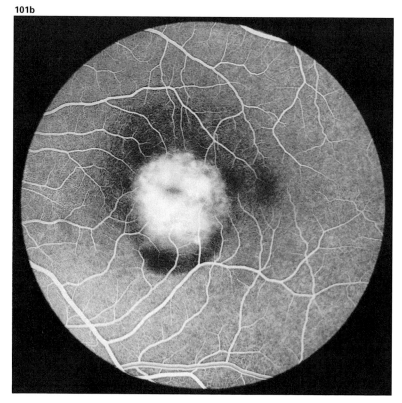

101b

101 Best's vitelliform dystrophy – pseudohypopyon stage. (**a**) An asymptomatic 31-year-old man was referred for investigation of his maculopathy. His mother had been found to have macular degeneration in her mid-forties. His uncle was also affected but was still able to drive a car. (**b**) Most of the lesion visible on the colour photograph demonstrates an intense patchy hyperfluorescence, although there is relative hypofluorescence corresponding to the fluid level. There is a ring of masking of choroidal fluorescence around the lesion.

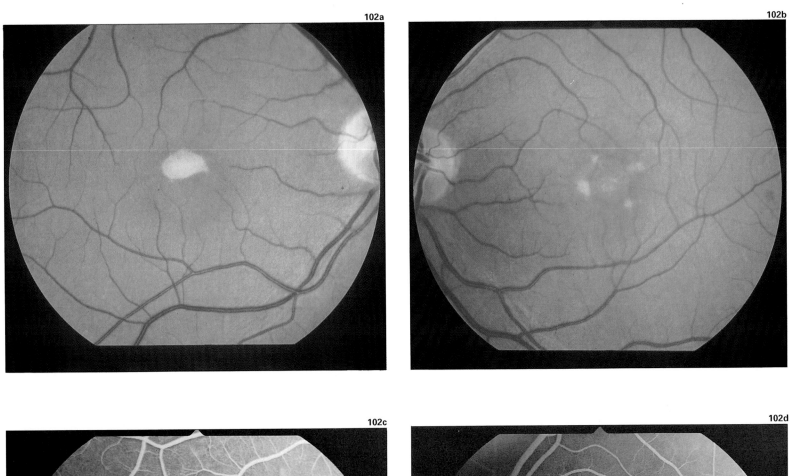

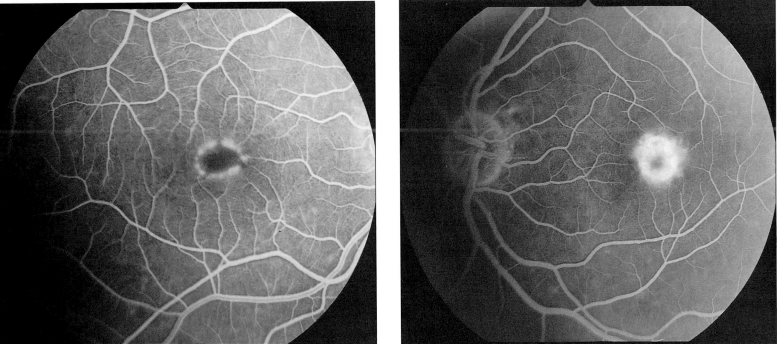

102 Adult onset foveovitelliform dystrophy. (**a,b**) A 44-year-old man presented with visual acuities 6/12, 6/36. (**c**) Right eye: There is masking by the yellow material. (**d**) On the left there is hyperfluorescence corresponding with a circular patch of atrophy.

Bibliography

Gass JDM. *Stereoscopic atlas of macular diseases*. St Louis: Mosby, 1987; Chapter 5 (Heredodystrophic disorders affecting the pigment epithelium and retina).

Ryan SJ. *Retina*. St Louis: Mosby, 1989; Chapter 20 (Retinitis pigmentosa and allied disorders) and Chapter 69 (Macular dystrophies).

9 The optic disc

Fluorescein angiographic studies have contributed to the understanding of the circulation at the optic nerve head, and to some of the pathological processes involved in open angle glaucoma and ischaemia of the optic nerve head. There is some evidence that filling defects of the disc are associated with glaucomatous cupping and correlate with field loss, and that there may be abnormalities in the circulation of the peripapillary choroid. However, there is overlap with normal appearances, and other non-invasive methods for diagnosis and monitoring of glaucoma are readily available.

In the early days of fluorescein angiography, the investigation was much used for the assessment of optic disc swelling, particularly to distinguish between appearances due to pathological swelling and so-called pseudopapilloedema. Now that less invasive radiological techniques such as computerized tomography (CT) and magnetic resonance imaging (MRI) are available, disc angiography is used less as a diagnostic aid. It remains useful in some cases where there is doubt about the presence of disc oedema.

Papilloedema

Clinical signs In papilloedema, disc swelling due to raised intracranial pressure, the disc is raised above the retinal surface. Haemorrhages and cotton wool spots are often seen and the prepapillary capillaries are dilated. Some vessels traversing the optic nerve head may be buried over part of their course, and venous pulsation is usually absent. Visual field examination shows an enlarged blind spot, but unless optic atrophy has developed, central visual acuity is preserved.

Angiographic appearances Angiography in established papilloedema shows dilatation of the prepapillary capillary plexus with leakage of dye. The disc becomes intensely hyperfluorescent with extension of the fluorescence beyond the disc boundaries (**103**).

There is no fluorescence beyond the margins of the disc, and leakage is sometimes difficult to detect in very early papilloedema. In longstanding papilloedema, refractile bodies can be misinterpreted as drusen. An equivocal angiogram with signs or symptoms of raised intracranial pressure suggests the need for further investigations.

Drusen of the optic nerve head

Clinical findings Drusen may be exposed, partly exposed or buried. When exposed, they have a craggy, yellow, irregular appearance and diagnosis is rarely a problem. When buried, the optic nerve head is smoothly elevated which may give rise to confusion with pathological swelling. This appearance poses problems, particularly in children and young people, before the drusen become exposed. Additional signs such as venous pulsation and anomalous vessel patterns, together with absence of dilatation of the prepapillary plexus and of a physiological cup, are enough to confirm the diagnosis. An examination of the parents is useful as disc drusen are often inherited.

Buried drusen are occasionally associated with deep haemorrhages, but there are no cotton wool spots. The discs are often small and have an irregular border with surrounding retinal pigment epithelial defects. A variety of associated field defects, including enlargement of the blind spot, arcuate scotomas, inferior nasal defects and generalized constriction, have been reported.

Angiographic appearances When exposed, drusen deposits show autofluorescence—they are fluorescent in the exciting blue beam before dye is injected (**104**). After injection, there is gradual uptake of dye and the disc remains fluorescent in the late pictures. The fluorescence is irregular in intensity and has a well-defined margin corresponding with the margin of the disc, except where there are overlying drusen. Dye does not enter the surrounding retina as it does in papilloedema. Anomalous vascular patterns, with increased numbers of major vessels on the disc, anomalous branching with trifurcations and increased tortuosity, are often found in association with disc drusen. Buried drusen (**105**) do not autofluoresce; angiographic appearances are otherwise similar.

Other causes of pseudopapilloedema

Hypermetropic discs and other congenital malformations may sometimes be confused with pathological swelling. A careful clinical examination is usually all that is required but, if necessary, an angiogram will confirm the absence of abnormal capillaries and leakage.

Papillitis

Localized swelling of the optic nerve head associated with marked visual deterioration and an afferent pupillary defect is traditionally termed papillitis or neuritis, although in many cases there is no evidence that an inflammatory process is involved. The swelling is indistinguishable, both clinically and on fluorescein angiography, from that seen in papilloedema. However, the symptoms and associated signs make the distinction easy. Angiography shows dilated capillaries with leakage of dye as seen with papilloedema, although there may occasionally be other features specific to the particular disorder (**106**).

Papillitis with uveitis The angiogram shows additional features depending on the cause of inflammation. Associated findings are macular oedema and scattered foci of leakage from retinal vessels over the posterior pole (see **89,97**). There may be evidence of vasculitis or focal inflammatory chorioretinal lesions, and of systemic disease, for example sarcoidosis (see **93**).

Papillitis associated with demyelinating disease There are no specific findings in this condition and differentiation is based on the clinical history, particularly the loss of central vision. Accompanying signs of inflammation, including uveitis, vitritis and vasculitis, have all been documented in multiple sclerosis. Difficulties in diagnosis arise where the history is atypical or the condition is bilateral.

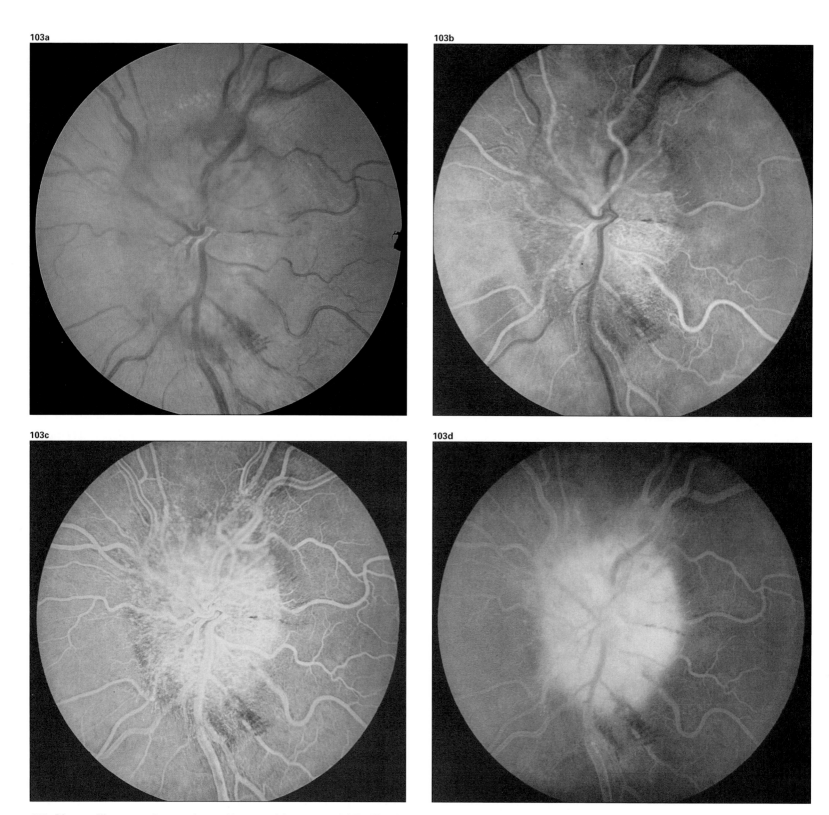

103 Disc swelling secondary to elevated intracranial pressure. (**a**) Papilloedema in a patient with acoustic neuroma. (**b**) Early pictures show dilated prepapillary capillaries. Patches of hypofluorescence correspond to haemorrhages. Because of the elevation of the disc, the upper part is not in focus. (**c**) The disc becomes more intensely hyperfluorescent as dye leaks from the capillaries. (**d**) Only faint hyperfluorescence is seen in the retinal vessels in the residual pictures, but the disc remains hyperfluorescent, with the the hyperfluorescence extending beyond its borders, characteristically above and below. The edges of the hyperfluorescent area are indistinct.

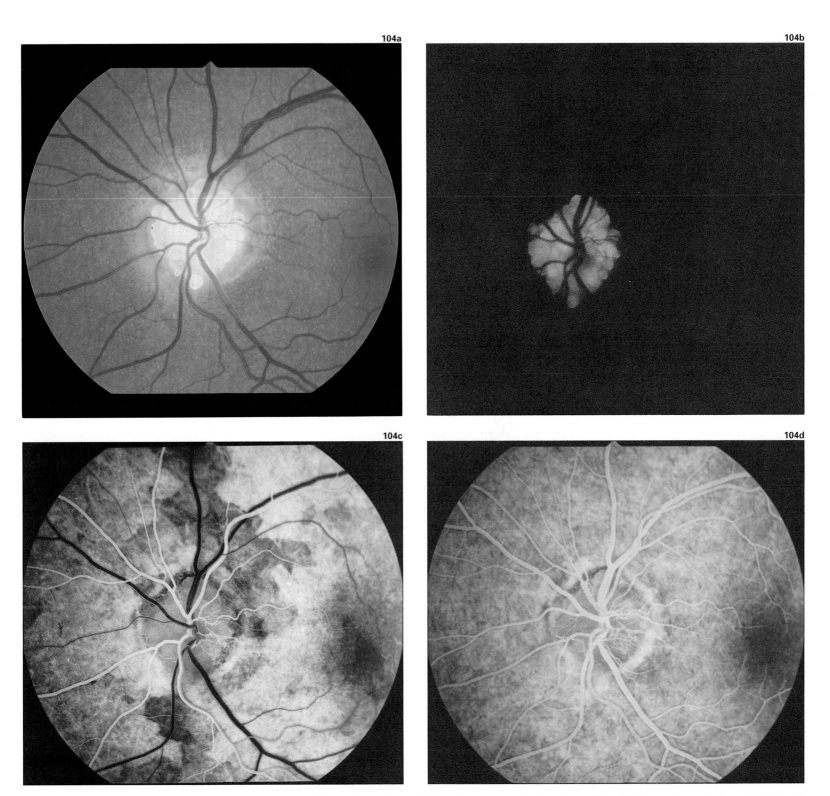

104 Disc drusen. (**a**) A 28-year-old man was noted by his optician to have abnormal discs. There was no family history. Visual fields were irregularly constricted and the visual acuity was 6/12, 6/9. (**b**) The discs are autofluorescent. This picture was taken before the injection of dye. (**c**) Early picture showing patchy choroidal filling within the normal range. The prepapillary capillaries show a normal pattern. (**d**) There is no leakage from the disc capillaries and the boundaries remain distinct. The hyperfluorescent halo around the the disc and the partial hypofluorescent ring correspond to pallor and increased pigmentation, respectively, on the colour picture. Choroidal filling is normal.

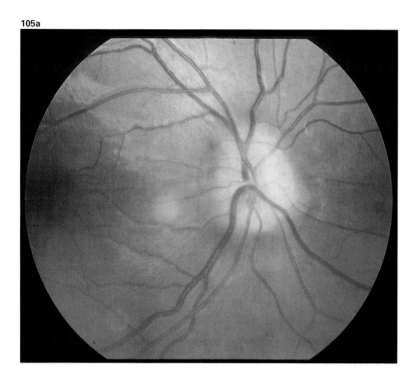

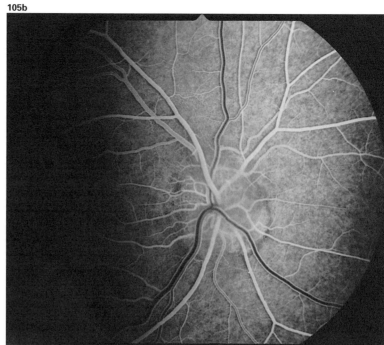

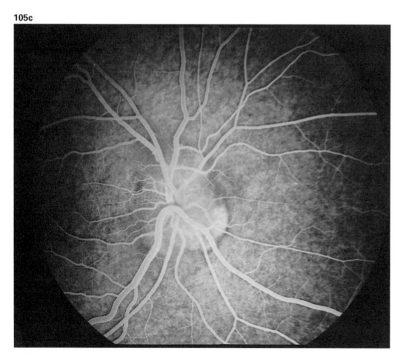

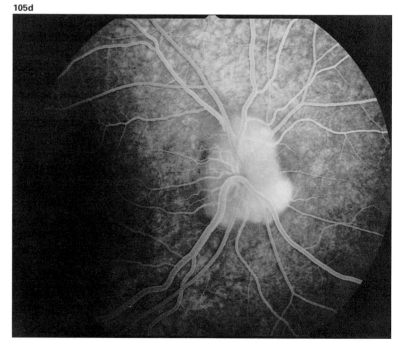

105 Disc drusen. (**a**) This 14-year-old boy was found to have elevated optic discs. There were no visual symptoms. His mother was known to have optic disc drusen. (**b**) Early venous phase. Note the slight loss of focus in the anterior plane of the disc due to its elevation. Early staining is observed. (**c**) The disc is hyperfluorescent with an irregular border. There is no evidence of leakage from normal calibre prepapillary capillaries. (**d**) The disc remains hyperfluorescent in the residual phase, in this case now six minutes after the injection of dye. The hyperfluorescence is of uneven intensity. The boundary of the hyperfluorescent area has not altered during the course of the angiogram.

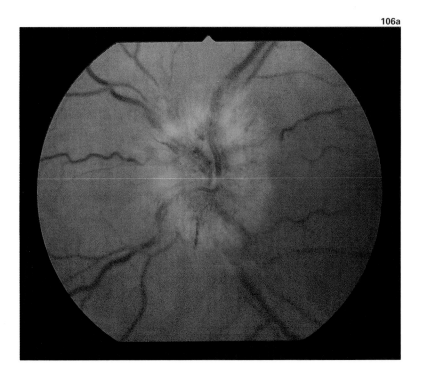

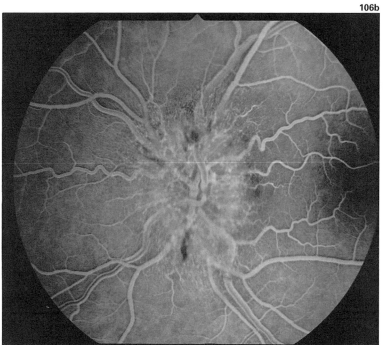

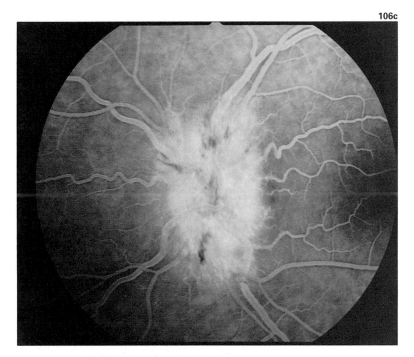

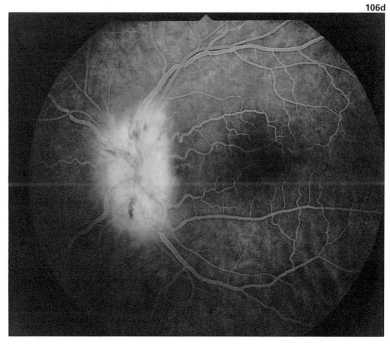

106 Papillitis. (**a**) An otherwise healthy 60-year-old man presented with sudden unilateral visual loss and an afferent pupillary defect. His visual acuity was 6/6, but a quadrantic field defect was detected. An ischaemic cause for his papillitis is suspected, but no obvious filling defect of the disc or peripapillary choroid was demonstrated. (**b**) Angiography demonstrated dilated and telangiectatic prepapillary capillaries. (**c**) There is increased leakage of dye from the disc. (**d**) The disc remains hyperfluorescent in the late pictures. The hyperfluorescent area has a 'fuzzy' border and extends beyond the normal disc boundary.

Ischaemic papillitis Angiography is sometimes helpful in distinguishing ischaemia of the optic nerve head from other causes of pathological disc swelling. Filling defects of the disc and delay in filling of the peripapillary choroid are sometimes detected (**107**). Where a portion of the disc is swollen with corresponding altitudinal or arcuate field loss, a filling defect of the affected section of the disc is usually demonstrated. If the whole disc is involved such filling defects are difficult to detect. However, diagnosis is usually based on the history and age of the patient. In cases of giant cell arteritis, the symptoms, together with a raised erythrocyte sedimentation rate or plasma viscosity, usually render further investigation superfluous; confirmation, if required, is made on the basis of temporal artery biopsy.

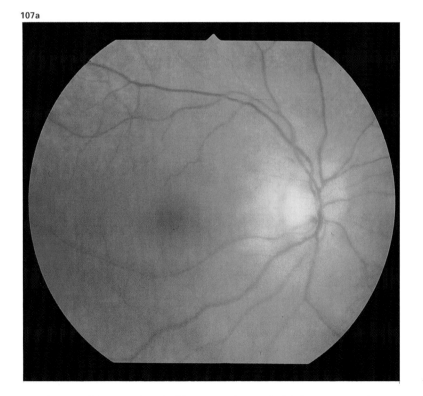

107a

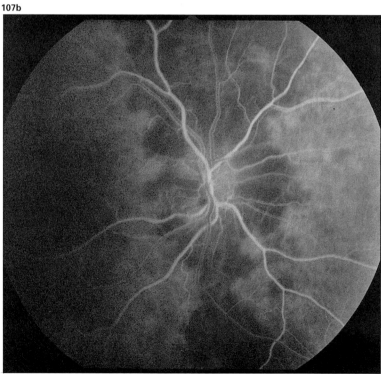

107b

107 Disc swelling associated with temporal arteritis. (**a**) An 80-year-old woman had been feeling unwell with headache, scalp hyperaesthesia, jaw claudication and intermittent clouding of her right vision. Her erythrocyte sedimentation rate was 88mm per hour and a temporal artery biopsy was positive. Treatment with systemic steroids was started, but a few days later her right visual acuity deteriorated rapidly until she could no longer perceive light with that eye. An angiogram was performed. (**b**) The choroidal filling defect noted in this early picture could be within the normal range at this stage, but it persists much longer than would be expected.

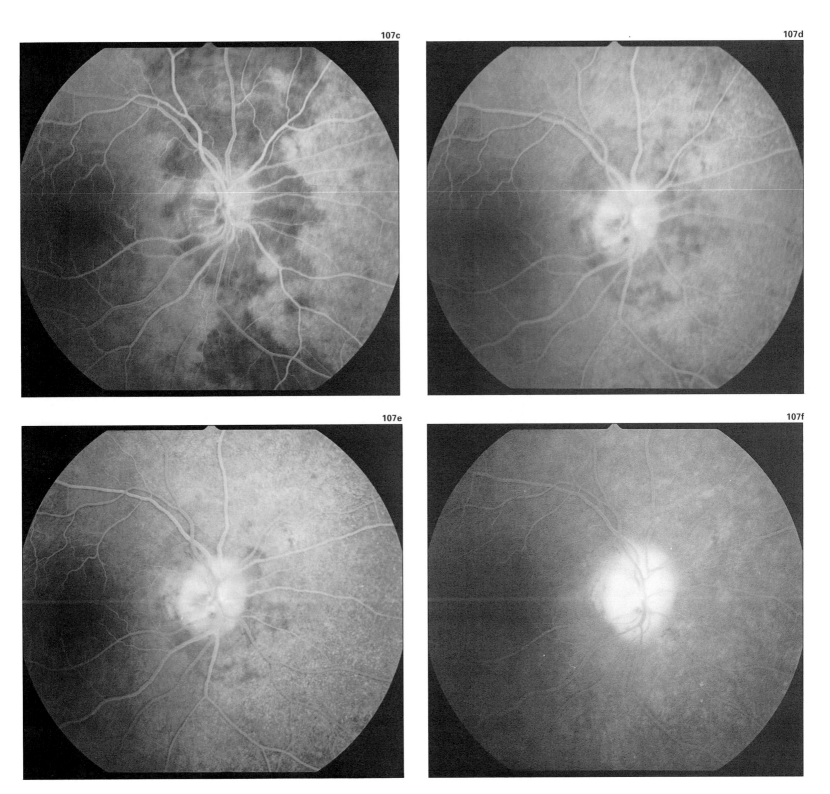

107 Disc swelling associated with temporal arteritis (contd). (**c,d,e**). There is a persistent filling defect on the temporal side of the disc. (**f**) The late picture shows an intensely fluorescent disc with indistinct borders.

Optic disc pits

An optic disc pit is an uncommon abnormality of the optic nerve head, thought to be due to incomplete closure of the embryonic fissure. Other associated abnormalities include colobomata of the disc and retina. There is a small, deep, circular depression in the surface of the disc and a corresponding field defect is often detected. Optic disc pits are also associated with a serous elevation of the retina at the macula. The mechanism by which macular changes develop is unclear.

On angiography the pit is hypofluorescent in the early frames, and sometimes shows late staining. There seems to be a higher incidence of late hyperfluorescence in pits associated with macular elevation, but no perfusion of dye into the subretinal fluid is detectable (**108**).

108a

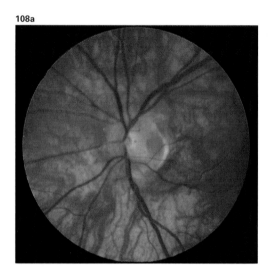

108b

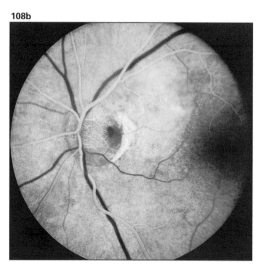

108c

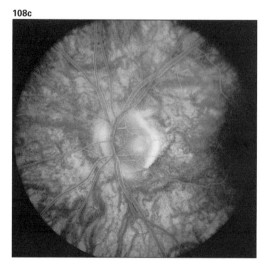

108 Optic disc pit. (**a**) A 20-year-old woman was referred because of the appearance of her left optic disc. She was asymptomatic, but her left visual acuity was 6/9 and a shallow serous macular detachment was noted. (**b**) The optic disc pit is hypofluorescent in the early pictures. (**c**) Late photograph demonstrating staining of the pit.

Bibliography

Cartlidge NEF, Ng RCY, Tilley PJB. Dilemma of the swollen optic disc: a fluorescein retinal angiography study. *Br J Ophthalmol* 1977;**61**:385–9.

Gass JDM. *Stereoscopic Atlas of Macular Disorders*.St Louis: Mosby, 1987; Chapter 13 (Optic nerve diseases that may masquerade as macular diseases).

Hayreh SS. Recent advances in fluorescein fundus angiography. *Br J Ophthalmol* 1974;**58**:391–412.

Kelley JS. Autofluorescence of drusen of the optic nerve head. *Arch Ophthalmol* 1974;**92**:263–4.

Rosenberg MA, Savino PJ, Glaser JS. A clinical analysis of pseudopapilledema. *Arch Ophthalmol* 1979;**97**:65–70.

Ryan SJ. *Retina*. St Louis: Mosby, 1989; Chapter 114 (Optic disc pits and associated serous macular detachment) and Chapter 115 (Optic nerve drusen).

Sanders MD, ffytche TJ. Fluorescein angiography in the diagnosis of drusen of the disc. *Trans Ophthalmol Soc UK* 1967;**87**:457–68.

Sanders MD, Sennhenn RH. Differential diagnosis of unilateral optic disc oedema. *Trans Ophthalmol Soc UK* 1980;**100**:123–31.

Spaeth GL. Fluorescein angiography: its contribution towards understanding the mechanisms of visual loss in glaucoma. *Trans Am Ophthalmol Soc* 1975;**73**:491–553.

10 *Fundus tumours*

The differential diagnosis of tumours of the fundus continues to challenge the diagnostic skills of the clinician. The discovery of a choroidal malignant melanoma no longer results automatically in enucleation, and other options include continuing observation (for growth), radiotherapy, local excision and photocoagulation. However, the distinction between this life-threatening condition and benign fundus tumours remains crucial and decisions regarding management depend on an accurate diagnosis.

Fluorescein angiography is a standard investigation in the assessment of ocular tumours, and the angiographic features are in many cases characteristic. However, a reliance on angiography to establish a diagnosis of melanoma would be unwise as the appearance may be mimicked by other tumours; other tests, including visual fields and ultrasound examination, should also be employed. A masked study by experienced observers showed that only 50% of melanomas could be diagnosed on the basis of angiography alone.

Malignant choroidal melanoma

Often there is little doubt about the clinical diagnosis when a large, elevated, pigmented lesion of characteristic appearance is seen. However, difficulties arise in cases where the tumour is small, amelanotic or very densely pigmented, or in the presence of overlying degenerative changes of the retinal pigment epithelium and neuroretina.

Choroidal melanomas tend to be irregularly hyperfluorescent as a result of their vascularity and changes in the overlying pigment epithelium and neuroretina. Angiography demonstrates the abnormal tumour vessels which are choroidal in origin and permeable to fluorescein (**109**). The tumour is sometimes hypofluorescent in the early frames, but in other cases it fluoresces early. During the course of the angiogram, the fluorescence spreads to obscure the vascular pattern and becomes intense in the late pictures. However, densely pig-

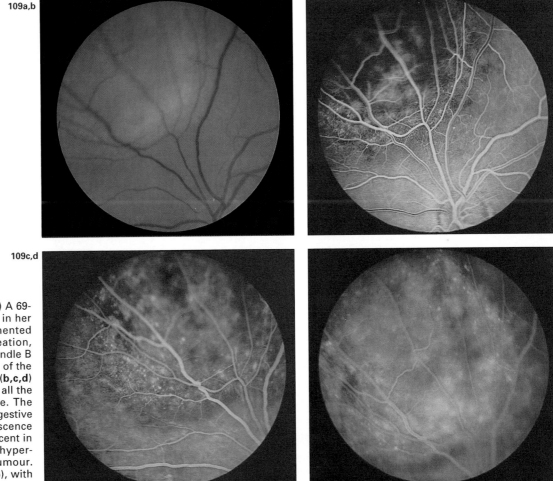

109a,b

109c,d

109 Malignant melanoma of the choroid. (**a**) A 69-year-old woman had noticed flashing lights in her left field of vision. A large, elevated, pigmented tumour was discovered. Following enucleation, histological examination demonstrated a spindle B choroidal melanoma. There was no invasion of the sclera, Bruch's membrane or optic nerve. (**b,c,d**) Because of the thickness of the tumour, not all the tumour is sharply in focus at any one time. The lesion shows patchy hyperfluorescence suggestive of an intrinsic circulation. The hyperfluorescence spreads and the tumour is intensely fluorescent in the late picture. There are many small hyperfluorescent dots around the edges of the tumour. Dilatation of retinal capillaries is seen in (**b**), with leakage later.

119

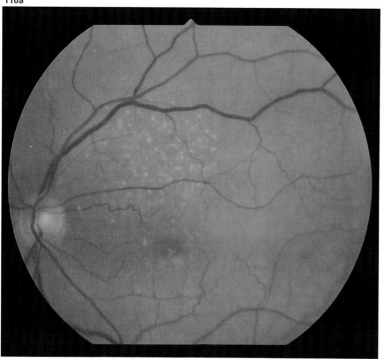

110a

mented tumours may remain hypofluorescent throughout the angiographic sequence, and associated haemorrhage also causes masking. In some malignant melanomas, large vessels are seen within the tumour. These have been interpreted as an intrinsic or 'double' circulation.

The pattern and intensity of fluorescence depends to a great extent on the integrity of the overlying pigment epithelium, neuroretina and Bruch's membrane. The pigment epithelium may be deficient in some places, with atrophy over and around the tumour, and clumped and multilayered in others. Accumulation of orange lipofuscin deposits is a frequent finding. An overlying serous detachment of the neuroretina with intraretinal oedema is sometimes a feature. It is important to realise that secondary degeneration is not specific to malignant melanoma and may occur over other large benign tumours.

Angiography sometimes shows a pattern of small hyperfluorescent spots which change in size and number during the evolution of the tumour. There is no agreement on the cause of this appearance.

Benign choroidal naevi

Benign choroidal naevi are a common incidental finding on routine clinical examination. In most cases the lesion is small and flat, but there may be some difficulty in differentiating bulky naevi from small malignant melanomas. In such patients, angiography is often helpful.

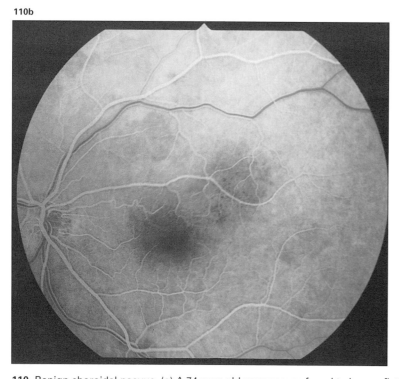

110b

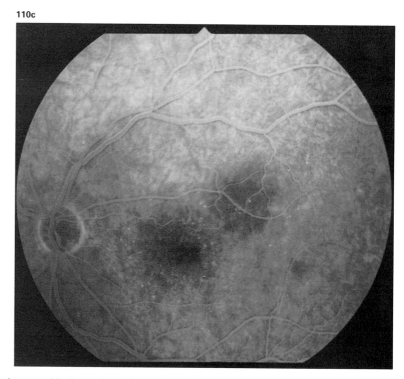

110c

110 Benign choroidal naevus. (**a**) A 74-year-old woman was found to have a flat pigmented lesion at her left posterior pole. She was asymptomatic with a visual acuity of 6/6, N 5. (**b,c**) The lesion is hypofluorescent with masking of the underlying choroid. A few small drusen overly it.

Angiographic appearance Most naevi are hypofluorescent, particularly in the early part of the transit (**110**). The choriocapillaris is usually intact and the later pictures are therefore often normal, although the hypofluorescence may persist. A small proportion are amelanotic and hyperfluorescent without demonstrating an abnormal circulation. Overlying degenerative changes of the pigment epithelium and neuroretina have been described, though not as commonly as in malignant tumours. Overlying drusen are a more frequent finding with benign rather than malignant melanomas.

Focal congenital abnormalities of the retinal pigment epithelium

These include retinal pigment hypertrophy, retinal pigment epithelial hyperplasia, combined hamartoma of the pigment epithelium and retina and congenital albinotic and amelanotic naevi of the pigment epithelium. They are rare, and only the first two are described in more detail.

Retinal pigment epithelial hypertrophy This benign lesion is flat, highly pigmented, and has a characteristic well-defined border. Angiography shows hypofluorescence corresponding to the pigmented area and a normal overlying retinal vascular pattern, although sometimes there may be capillary irregularities (**111**). Larger and older lesions have a tendency to develop patches of hypopigmentation.

The condition known as 'bear tracks' (groups of pigmented patches reminiscent of a bear's paw prints in the snow) is a rare manifestation of retinal pigment epithelial hypertrophy.

Retinal pigment epithelial hyperplasia Retinal pigment epithelial hyperplasia occurring in response to inflammation or trauma is a common condition. Congenital pigment epithelial hyperplasia is rare. The lesion is black and nodular, arising from the pigment epithelium and extending into the neuroretina. Angiography demonstrates masking, and, unlike pigment epithelial hypertrophy, no retinal vessels are visible over the tumour.

111a

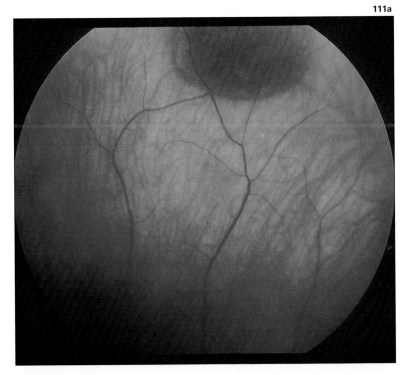

111b

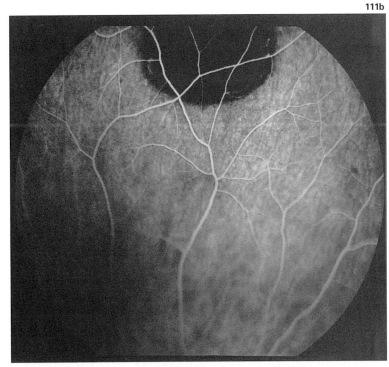

111 Pigment epithelial hypertrophy. (**a**) This young woman was referred for angiography because a malignant melanoma was suspected. The lesion is darkly pigmented and well demarcated, with the characteristic appearance of benign retinal pigment epithelial hypertrophy. (**b**) Dense hypofluorescence is caused by masking of the underlying choroid. Overlying retinal vessels are visible.

Metastatic tumours

Metastatic tumours, particularly from the breast, are not uncommon in the choroid; they rarely reach the attention of ophthalmologists as most patients with choroidal secondaries are in the terminal stages of cancer. Sometimes differentiation from malignant melanoma and other fundal tumours is difficult, but there are no characteristic findings on fluorescein angiography to aid diagnosis (**112**). Secondary tumours, however, have less tendency to develop a secondary circulation than malignant melanoma and therefore show vessels within the tumour less often. The early filling of large vascular spaces seen in choroidal haemangiomas is not a feature of secondary tumours.

Choroidal haemangioma

Choroidal haemangiomas are relatively rare benign tumours which affect both sexes equally. A diffuse form is found in the Sturge–Weber syndrome, but it is the discrete form which is likely to cause problems with diagnosis.

Discrete haemangiomas tend to have a reddish appearance with pale streaks. The overlying retina may show cystic degeneration and a localized accumulation of subretinal fluid. Overlying hyperplasia of the pigment epithelium can make differentiation from malignant melanomas difficult; under these circumstances, angiography and ultrasound examination are often helpful.

Choroidal haemangiomas have an abnormal pattern of large vascular channels which is characteristically seen early on an angiogram, before the filling of retinal arterioles. During the course of the angiogram there is diffuse and irregular leakage over the tumour. In the late pictures a pattern of cystic spaces is demonstrated in the overlying retina (**113**). The early transit appearances, while not pathognomonic, are highly suggestive of a choroidal haemangioma. However, all these angiographic findings have been described with malignant melanoma and it may be impossible to distinguish some haemangiomas from malignant melanomas on the basis of fluorescein angiography alone.

Choroidal osteoma

Choroidal osteomas are found most frequently in adult white women. They are usually juxtapapillary and pale yellow or orange in colour, with a well-defined border. Small vascular networks are seen on the surface. An overlying pattern of mottled depigmentation may suggest malignant melanoma. The lesions are often asymptomatic when first discovered, but a significant proportion of patients subsequently develops visual loss as a result of subretinal neovascularization.

Angiography shows early patchy hyperfluorescence and late staining. The choroidal vascular tufts are demonstrated early, and then fade. Subretinal neovascularization is characterized by persistent hyperfluorescence and leakage of dye (**114**).

Diagnosis is confirmed by ultrasonography and computerized tomography, which demonstrate the presence of bone within the lesion.

112a,b,c

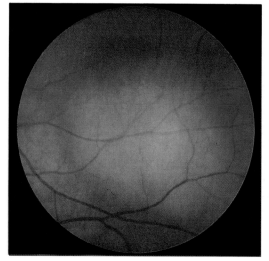 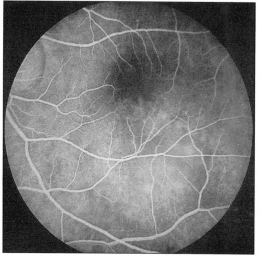 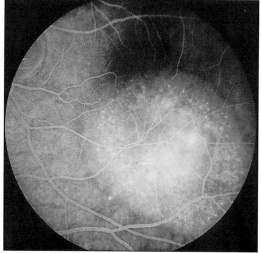

112 Choroidal metastasis. (**a**) A metastasis from a carcinoma of the breast. (**b,c**) The tumour shows patchy hyperfluorescence. Hyperfluorescent dots surround it in the late pictures. There is no obvious secondary circulation, but it would be difficult to differentiate it from a malignant melanoma on angiography alone.

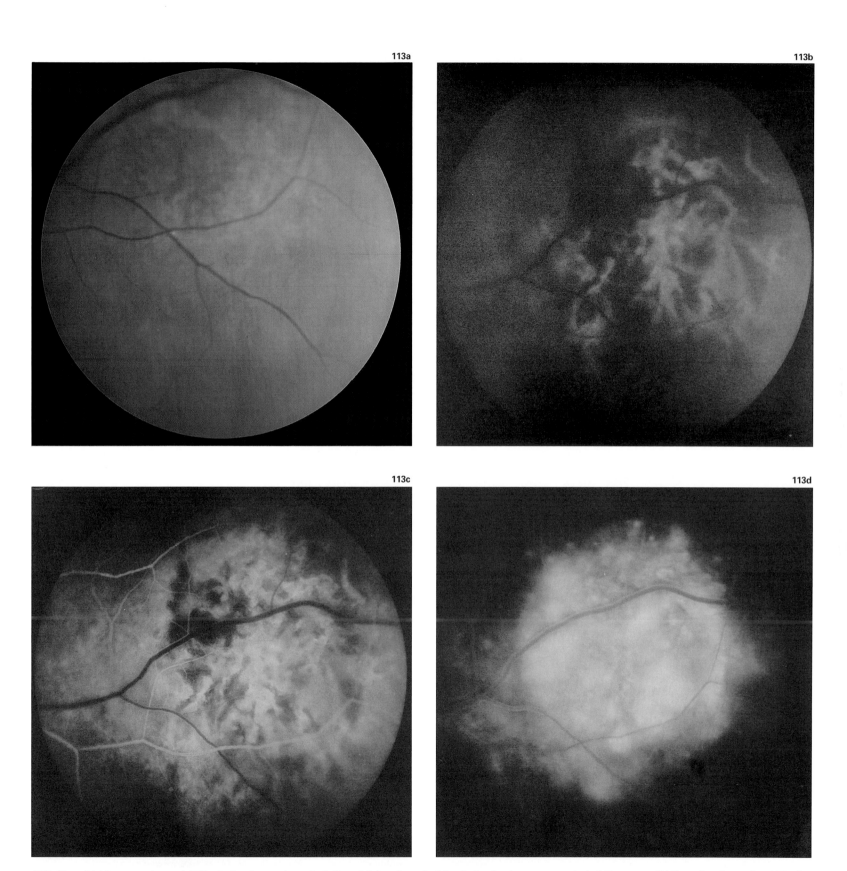

113 Choroidal haemangioma. (**a**) The lesion has a characteristic reddish colour. It did not alter in size over a period of five years. (**b**) Vascular channels within the tumour are seen in the very earliest frame as the choroid starts to fill, before there is any dye in the retinal vessels. (**c,d**) During the course of the angiogram the entire lesion becomes hyperfluorescent. The late picture shows large patches of persisting fluorescence, suggesting pooling of dye.

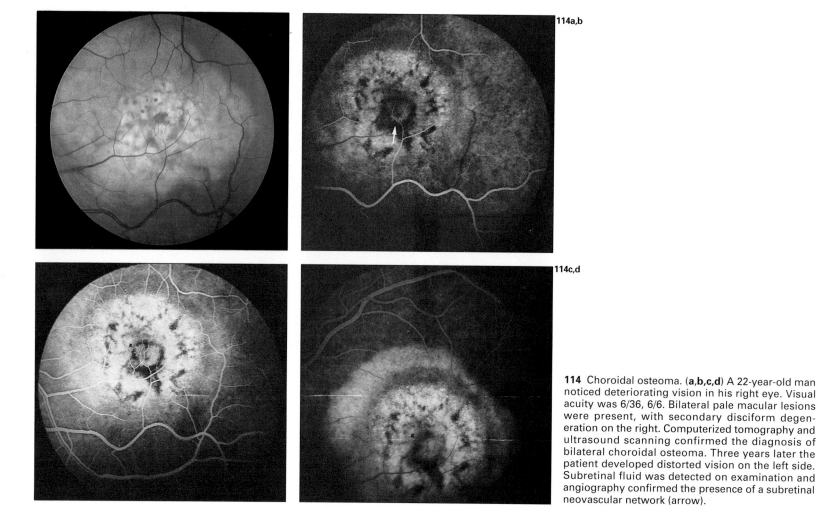

114 Choroidal osteoma. (**a,b,c,d**) A 22-year-old man noticed deteriorating vision in his right eye. Visual acuity was 6/36, 6/6. Bilateral pale macular lesions were present, with secondary disciform degeneration on the right. Computerized tomography and ultrasound scanning confirmed the diagnosis of bilateral choroidal osteoma. Three years later the patient developed distorted vision on the left side. Subretinal fluid was detected on examination and angiography confirmed the presence of a subretinal neovascular network (arrow).

Bibliography

Bloom PA, Ferris JD, Laidlaw DAH, Goddard PR. Magnetic resonance imaging: Diverse appearances of uveal malignant melanomas. *Arch Ophthalmol* 1992;**110**:1105–11.

Collaborative Ocular Melanoma Study Group. Accuracy of diagnosis of choroidal melanomas in the collaborative ocular melanoma study. *Arch Ophthalmol* 1990;**108**:1268–73.

Davis DL, Robertson DM. Fluorescein angiography of metastatic choroidal tumours. *Arch Ophthalmol* 1973;**89**:97–9.

Ferry AP. Lesions mistaken for malignant melanoma of the posterior uvea: a clinicopathological analysis of 100 cases with ophthalmologically visible lesions. *Arch Ophthalmol* 1964;**72**:463–7.

Gass JDM. *Stereoscopic Atlas of Macular Diseases*. St Louis: Mosby, 1987; Chapter 3 (Diseases causing choroidal exudative and hemorrhagic localised [disciform] detachment of the retinal and pigment epithelium) and Chapter 10 (Retinal and pigment epithelial hamartomas).

Gass JDM. Focal congenital anomalies of the retinal pigment epithelium. *Eye* 1989;**3**:1–18.

Gass JDM, Guerry RK, Jack RL, Harris G. Choroidal osteoma. *Arch Ophthalmol* 1978;**96**:428–35.

Hayreh SS. Choroidal melanomata. Fluorescence angiographic and histopathological study. *Brit J Ophthalmol* 1970;**54**:145–60.

Joffe L, Shields JA, Fitzgerald JR. Osseous choristoma of the choroid. *Arch Ophthalmol* 1978;**96**:1809.

Pettit TH, Barton A, Foos RY, Christensen RE. Fluorescein angiography of choroidal melanomas. *Arch Ophthalmol* 1970;**83**:27–38.

Purcell JJ, Shields JA. Hypertrophy with hyperpigmentation of the retinal pigment epithelium. *Arch Ophthalmol* 1975;**93**:1122–6.

Robertson DM, Campbell RJ. Errors in the diagnosis of malignant melanoma of the choroid. *Am J Ophthalmol* 1979;**87**:269–75.

Ryan SJ. *Retina*. St Louis: Mosby, 1989; Chapter 39 (Diagnosis of choroidal melanoma), Chapter 50 (Choroidal metastasis), Chapter 51 (Choroidal osteoma) and Chapter 52 (Choroidal hemangioma).

Shields JA. Lesions simulating malignant melanoma of the posterior uvea. *Arch Ophthalmol* 1973;**89**:466–71.

Shields JA, Annesley WH Jr, Totino JA. Nonfluorescent malignant melanoma of the choroid diagnosed with the radioactive phosphorus uptake test. *Am J Ophthalmol* 1975;**79**:634–40.

11 Advances in fundus fluorescein angiography

Fluorescein angiography has stood the test of time and remains an essential investigation in the study of fundus disorders. The technique is relatively safe, convenient, and inexpensive—it is unlikely to be superseded in the near future.

Recent technological advances, however, particularly in laser and computer systems, promise improvements in safety and patient acceptability, and in the storage, analysis and retrieval of results.

Processing, storage and retrieval systems

The storage and retrieval of angiograms pose problems which have been resolved in different ways by different departments. Negatives are easily lost or damaged when stored in the patients' notes. When kept in a central filing area, they are bulky and vulnerable to damage through frequent handling. Filing and retrieval are labour-intensive. In some departments, positive transparencies or prints are stored in patients' records, but quality is lost in the reproduction and the process is time-consuming and expensive.

Many departments provide a reporting service. A room is equipped with light screens, magnifying lenses and projectors, and a clinician with particular expertise examines all the angiograms and provides a written report. Nevertheless, it is still often necessary to examine the angiogram in the consulting room or before treatment.

Digitization and computerization of the angiographic images promise an answer to these problems in the future. Since each point on a frame from a fluorescein angiogram can be characterized by its position and its intensity, it can be digitized. The information is stored on computer and can later be analysed, compared with previous records, retrieved as necessary and transmitted readily to other locations. Such systems, which are in development, have potential in monitoring disease progress and allowing comparison with reference photographs. However, they do not as yet match the resolution of a conventional negative.

Video angiography

Although not generally available, video angiography is used routinely in some centres as an alternative to standard angiography.

The most obvious advantage of the technique is that it provides a dynamic image. The earliest appearance of dye in the vasculature and the phases of circulation can be more precisely recorded. The image is recorded on video tape and can therefore be retrieved immediately after the angiogram, avoiding the delay inherent in photographic film processing. The video tape can be replayed, slowed down or frozen, and the images transmitted to other workstations. Projection or magnification systems are not required for interpretation.

The resolution of video angiograms, however, is not as good as that of conventional sequential angiography. The equipment is complex and costly, and the angiogram can be viewed only where a monitor and video system are available for playback. Hard copies are obtainable, but do not match the quality of standard negatives.

The scanning laser ophthalmoscope

The scanning laser ophthalmoscope is a recent development with the potential to revolutionize imaging in ophthalmology. However, the technique is still being developed and its present cost is high.

The laser ophthalmoscope has several advantages over conventional techniques. A low level of retinal irradiance is required to obtain an image. The laser scans the fundus, illuminating a tiny area at a time, and the high collimation of the beam means that sufficient illumination is obtained through a small aperture. Light detectors, far more sensitive than photographic film, record the intensity of the reflected light; the information can be digitized and stored or displayed on a television screen. The average retinal irradiance required by the scanning laser ophthalmoscope is only 70 μW/cm compared with the 5,000 μW/cm required for viewing through the average fundus camera. The pupil does not have to be dilated and the examination is more comfortable, especially for photosensitive patients.

Lower doses of fluorescein are required for fluorescein angiography, and a dynamic recording is obtained with better resolution than a video recording using a fundus camera. There is less scattering of light by opacities in the media, and better images are obtained when these are present. It is now also possible to get a useful image with indocyanine green angiography using an infrared laser (see below).

Another advantage of the system is that it readily lends itself to advanced computer processing. Images can be analysed, stored, retrieved, compared and transmitted to other stations. Methods for analysing the three-dimensional structure of fundus features are being developed.

An important disadvantage of the laser scanning ophthalmoscope is that the image is monochromatic. Different wavelengths can be used to enhance different fundus features, but the colour images which are so familiar to ophthalmologists are yet to be achieved. This will cause initial problems in interpretation, and makes it less valuable as a teaching tool.

Indocyanine green angiography

Indocyanine green (ICG) has been proposed as an alternative to sodium fluorescein for fundus angiography. It has not gained general acceptance because of its low level of fluorescence compared to fluorescein (about 4%) and the difficulty of obtaining an acceptable image using conventional cameras. The laser scanning ophthalmoscope, using the infra-red wavelength, allows good resolution to be obtained, and it seems likely that the technique will be further developed and its full potential explored.

ICG is a water-soluble dye which fluoresces in the near infrared with a peak absorption at 805nm and a peak fluorescence at 835nm. It has certain advantages over fluorescein in angiography, particularly in the study of the choroid. The longer wavelengths are absorbed to a lesser extent by the pigment epithelium, permitting greater visibility of the choroidal layer. ICG is almost completely bound to plasma proteins and diffuses only slowly out of the choroidal capillaries. It promises to become a valuable tool for the study of the dynamics of the choroidal circulation and for detection of choroidal abnormalities.

It is likely that ICG will have a role in the management of exudative macular degeneration. Neovascular networks that are ill-defined on fluorescein angiography may be more precisely delineated with ICG. The reduction of leakage from the new vessel network may in some circumstances be a disadvantage, as fluorescein leakage is often an important diagnostic feature. Because of the increased visibility of the choroidal circulation, it may also be difficult to distinguish the network from the surrounding choroid and to determine the foveal centre. For the assessment of neovascular membranes with a view to treatment, therefore, a fluorescein angiogram is also necessary.

Bibliography

Destro M, Puliafito CA. Indocyanine green video angiography of choroidal neovascularisation. *Ophthalmol* 1989;**96**:846–53.

Klein GJ, Baumgartner RH, Flower RW. An image processing approach to characterising choroidal blood flow. *Invest Ophthalmol Vis Sci* 1990;**31**:629–37.

Meyer PAR, Fitzke FW. Computer assisted analysis of fluorescein videoangiograms. *Br J Ophthalmol* 1990;**74**:275–7.

Scheider A, Kaboth A, Neuhauser L. Detection of subretinal neovascular membranes with indocyanine green and an infrared scanning laser ophthalmoscope. *Am J Ophthalmol* 1992;**113**:45–51.

Scheider A, Schroedel C. High resolution indocyanine green angiography with a scanning laser ophthalmloscope (letter). *Am J Ophthalmol* 1989;**108**:458–9.

Seeley GW, Craine ER, Fryczkowski AW. Comparison of conventional fluorescein angiography film images with a cathode ray tube display. *Arch Ophthalmol* 1989;**107**:227–31.

Wolf S, Arend O, Toonen H *et al*. Retinal capillary blood flow measurement with a scanning laser ophthalmoscope. Preliminary results. *Ophthalmology* 1991;**98**:996–1000.

Woon WH, Fitzke FW, Chester GH *et al*. The scanning laser ophthalmoscope: Basic principles and applications. *J Ophthalmic Photography* 1999;**12**:17–23.

12 Fluorescein angiography of the anterior segment

Soon after the introduction of fundus fluorescein angiography, the technique was adpated for the investigation of disorders of the anterior segment. The first report, by Jensen and Lundbaek in 1968, described the iris and conjunctival vessels in diabetes mellitus. Since then a number of investigators have studied conjunctival, episcleral, iris and corneal vasculature. Much useful information has been obtained about the normal blood supply to the anterior segment and about the patterns of disturbance in disease. Although anterior segment angiography has an important place in research, it has not found the same widespread application as fundus angiography in the routine management of eye disease.

Method

The technique

The techniques used for fundus angiography are not directly applicable to angiography of the anterior segment. It has proved difficult to overcome the problems associated with the architecture and permeability of the anterior segment vasculature, the rapid dye transit time and the curved, reflecting surface of the eye.

The camera

Most investigators have employed modifications of the fundus camera or the photo-slit lamp. Others have used the binocular microscope, the single lens reflex camera or combinations of camera backs, lenses and light sources specifically designed for the purpose. The quality of angiograms has been restricted by problems with peripheral aberrations, limited depth of focus, reflections and difficulties in achieving correct levels of even illumination.

Early leakage – from normal conjunctival and episcleral vessels and from other anterior segment vasculature in disease – makes angiograms difficult to interpret, and a rapid sequence of photographs is essential during the early transit of the dye. This makes cine and video recordings particularly useful in anterior segment angiography.

115a

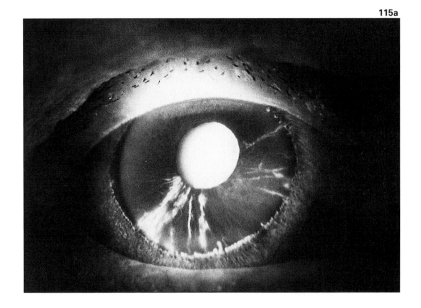

115b

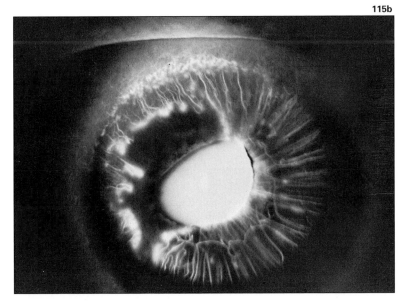

115c

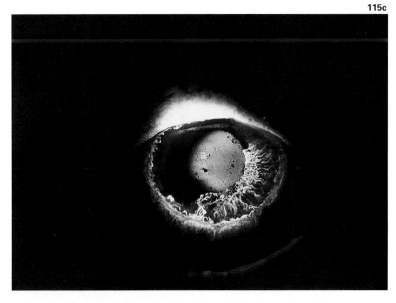

115 Anterior segment ischaemia. (**a**) Failure of iris perfusion following an attack of angle closure glaucoma. (**b,c**) Iris perfusion abnormalities in anterior segment ischaemia following retinal detachment surgery. Note the distorted pupil and leakage at vascular apices in (**b**). (Courtesy of Professor DL Easty.)

Most recently, the laser scanning ophthalmoscope has been modified to perform anterior segment fluorescein videoangiography. The system overcomes some of the disadvantages of sequential photography and conventional video techniques. The depth of focus is increased, producing a clear image over the entire field and reducing the effects of changes in position of the patient's eye or head. The coaxial beam gives a more even illumination and the low light levels are more comfortable for the patient. However, no video system achieves the spatial resolution of sequential photographic techniques.

The dye

The quantities and concentrations of dye used are the same as in fundus angiography, and good results have been reported with 5 ml of 10% or 20% fluorescein. More recently, low-dose angiography (0.6 ml of 20% fluorescein) has been used to demonstrate fine capillary detail. It is argued that at this level a higher proportion of fluorescein is bound to circulating albumin and its leakage from conjunctival and episcleral capillaries is reduced. More sensitive film and a modified development technique are required to compensate for the low levels of fluorescence.

The iris

Angiography of the normal iris demonstrates the radial pattern of arteries and veins. The sphincter capillary network is seen as a blush of fluorescence and details of individual capillaries are rarely demonstrated. The fluorescence of the vasculature is obscured by iris pigment and the technique is of limited value in patients with brown irides.

Abnormalities demonstrated by iris angiography include failure or delay in perfusion, dilatation of vessels, hyperpermeability and neovascularization. The filling pattern of normal iris vessels is highly variable and perfusion of different sectors tends to be asynchronous. It is often difficult to be certain, without reference to earlier photographs, whether perfusion delay in a particular case is pathological. Hyperpermeability should also be interpreted with care, as a degree of fluorescein leakage from iris vessels can be detected in some healthy patients, especially with increasing age.

Conditions causing ischaemia of the anterior segment have been studied using iris angiography (115). A delay in filling of sectors of iris has been demonstrated in both acute angle closure glaucoma and following detachment surgery. It is frequently found soon after surgery on the vertical rectus muscles, although the circulation usually recovers during the two weeks postoperatively. During attacks of acute ischaemia, vessels in the perfused part of the iris show dilatation and hyperpermeability, demonstrated by extensive leakage of dye.

Dilatation and leakage of radial vessels and leakage from areas of neovascularization have been described (116) following central retinal vein occlusion.

Other uses of iris angiography include assessment of iris tumours and the changes associated with open angle glaucoma.

The conjunctiva and episclera

Angiography of the conjunctiva and episclera has been complicated by the complex and multilayered vascular architecture, the wide range of appearances in the normal subject, the short transit time and the rapid extravasation of dye from normal vessels. Details of the episcleral vessels are often obscured by the overlying conjunctival plexus, and some veins fill before the arterial tree is completely perfused, thus making it difficult to determine in some cases whether a particular vessel is an artery or a vein. Low-dose techniques, and those using cine, video or laser technology, promise to answer many of the questions about normal anatomy which at present are unresolved or disputed.

Dye first appears in anterior ciliary arteries. Because of the rapid transit time it has been difficult to confirm whether the flow within them is centripetal, according to the traditional view, or centrifugal. Videoangiography can distinguish between arteries and veins by their flow characteristics and demonstrates that the anterior ciliary arteries may flow either towards or away from the limbus. This can be explained by the anatomy of the anterior segment blood supply: the long posterior ciliary and anterior ciliary arteries are joined by perforating trans-scleral vessels, forming trans-scleral arterial arcades (the sagittal arterial ring). The point at which the two circulations meet may lie at any position on this ring. The superficial anterior episcleral branches of the anterior ciliary artery run forward and anastomose with vessels from the adjacent anterior ciliary arteries to form an arte-

116 Iris neovascularization. Extensive leakage from iris new vessels. (Courtesy of Professor DL Easty.)

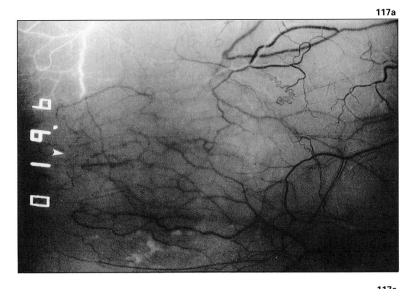

117a

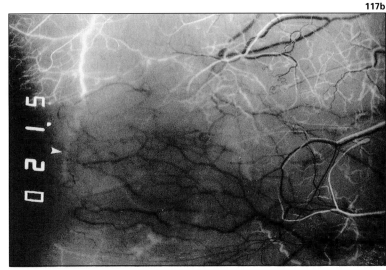

117b

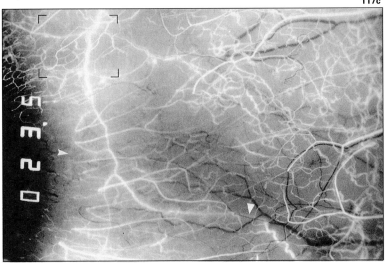

117c

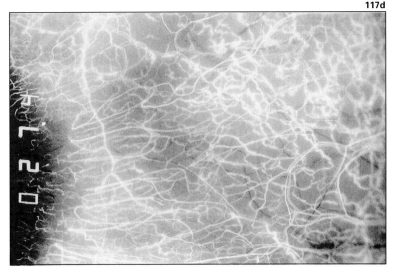

117d

117 Photographic low dose fluorescein angiography of the conjunctiva and episclera. Left temporal angiogram from a normal 32-year-old woman. (The time after injection is recorded on each frame.) (a) Fluorescein is first seen in an anterior ciliary artery branch that forms part of the anterior episcleral arterial circle. (b) After supplying a small territory of anterior conjunctiva, this vessel penetrates the sclera and continues at a deeper level (arrow). The posterior tarsal circulation begins to fill. (c) This fragment of the anterior episcleral arterial circle is completed by a superficial vessel that runs from the point of scleral penetration to an adjacent anterior ciliary artery. The vessel runs deep at the position shown by the arrow. From the episcleral arterial circle, anterior roots pass forward to the limbal reflection of the conjunctiva, where they feed the limbal arcades. They then loop back to supply the anterior conjunctiva. Note the characteristic, irregular net of episcleral capillaries, over which is arrayed the lace-like conjunctival plexus. The watershed zone between anterior ciliary and posterior tarsal contributions to the conjunctival plexus lies about 3mm from the limbus. This overlaps the region of late perfusion of the episcleral plexus. (d) Many radial anterior conjunctival vessels are veins, and in the posterior tarsal circulation veins accompany arteries. Leakage of fluorescein is minimal and never obscures anatomical detail. (e) Diagrammatic detail of the area bracketed in (c). Blood from the episcleral arterial circle (ec) is distributed to an anterior root, and thence into conjunctival arterioles (ca). Shunting of blood (arrowed) from an arteriole into an adjacent conjunctival venule (cv) explains the early perfusion of anterior conjunctival venules and the delayed fluorescence of the watershed zone (W). (Courtesy of Dr PAR Meyer.)

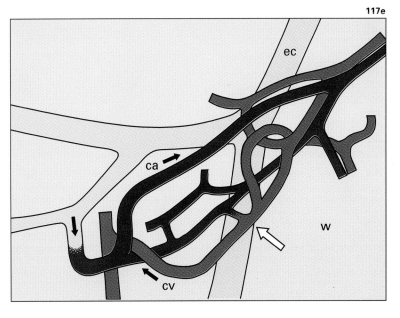

117e

rial circle. Branches from this circle supply the episcleral circulation, the anterior conjunctiva, the limbal arcades and contribute towards the circulation of the iris. The episcleral plexus is also fed posteriorly by vessels appearing at the level of the rectus muscle and the conjunctiva by branches of the posterior tarsal circulation (**117**).

There are wide variations in the normal circulation, both in architecture and in the timing of appearance and transit dye. It can therefore be difficult to distinguish a pathological abnormality. In inflammatory conditions, transit time is reduced further and profuse leakage occurs early, compounding the difficulties of detecting subtle abnormalities.

The main clinical application of conjunctival and episcleral angiography has been in the management of scleritis and sclerokeratitis (**118**). Slowing of the circulation and vascular closure are important indicators of severity, predicting necrotizing changes in the sclera or melting processes in the cornea. Demonstration of significant perfusion defects influences the choice of therapy with immunosuppressive agents. The area of abnormal circulation can be used as a guide to the extent of surgery required for scleral and/or corneal replacement in advanced cases with severe tissue destruction.

118a

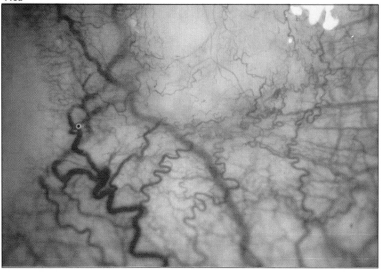

118b

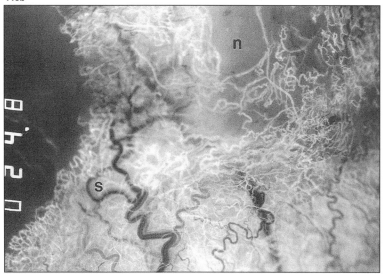

119

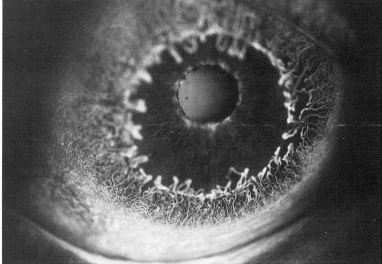

118 Scleritis. (**a**) Left temporal limbus in a 72-year-old man with necrotizing anterior scleritis complicating rheumatoid arthritis. (**b**) Low dose anterior segment fluorescein angiogram from the same field, 6 seconds after the first appearance of fluorescence. The conjunctival and episcleral circulations are absent over the necrotic sclera (n). There is intense leakage from damaged capillaries central to the lesion, but the limbal arcades have not yet become involved. An artery and vein (seen in silhouette) are confluent in a shunt (s) which bypasses the lesion. Perfusion of this circulation is delayed. The microcirculation in the lower part of the frame is anatomically normal, but the brisk perfusion and immediate leakage of fluorescein indicate inflammation. (Courtesy of Dr PAR Meyer.)

119 Corneal neovascularization following penetrating keratoplasty. Corneal new vessels extend through the corneal stroma into donor tissue. There is leakage of dye at the apices. (Courtesy of Professor DL Easty.)

The cornea

Fluorescein angiography has been used to study corneal neovascularization in different types of keratitis and following penetrating keratoplasty (**119,120**). Early pictures demonstrate the fine lacework pattern of the vasculature; later the pattern is obscured as fluorescein extravasates into the stroma.

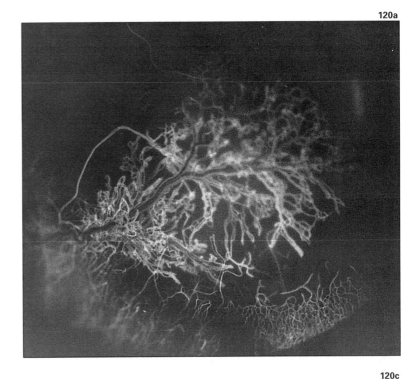

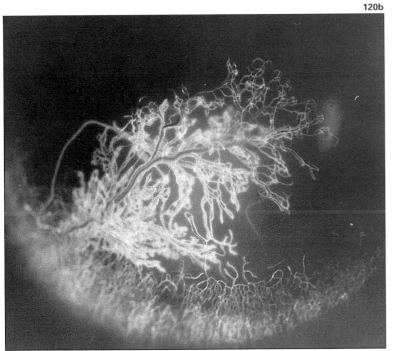

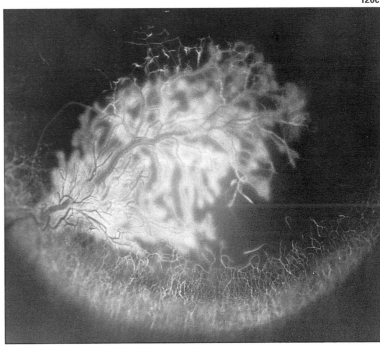

120 Corneal neovascularization in keratitis. (**a,b,c**) Angiographic sequence showing leash of neovascularization in exposure keratitis secondary to thyroid eye disease. Note leakage of dye in (**b**) leading to extensive hyperfluorescence within the corneal stroma in (**c**). (Courtesy of Professor DL Easty.)

Bibliography

Bron AJ, Easty DL. Fluorescein angiography of the globe and anterior segment. *Trans Ophthalmol Soc UK* 1970;**90**:339–67.

Chandler JW, Sewell JH, Kaufman HE. Anterior segment fluorescein angiography: A simple modification of the Zeiss stereo slit lamp camera. *Ann Ophthalmol* 1975;**7**:87–92.

Cheng H., Bron AJ, Easty D. A study of iris masses by fluorescein angiography. *Trans Ophthalmol Soc UK* 1971;**91**:199–205.

Chignell AH, Easty DL. Iris fluorescein photography following retinal detachment and in certain ocular ischaemic disorders. *Trans Ophthalmol Soc UK* 1971;**91**:243–59.

Easty DL, Chignell AH. Fluorescein angiography in anterior segment ischaemia. *Br J Ophthalmol* 1973;**57**:18–26.

Fetkenhour CL, Choromokos E. Anterior segment fluorescein angiography with a retinal fundus camera. *Arch Ophthalmol* 1978;**96**:711–13.

Jensen VA, Lundbaek K. Fluorescence angiography of the iris in recent and long-term diabetes. *Acta Ophthalmol* 1968;**46**:584–5.

Laatikainen, L. Preliminary report on effect of retinal panphotocoagulation on rubeosis iridis and neovascular glaucoma. *Br J Ophthalmol* 1977;**61**:278–284.

Marsh RJ, Ford SM. Cine photography and video recording of anterior segment fluorescein angiography. *Br J Ophthalmol* 1978;**62**:657–9.

Marsh RJ, Ford SM. Blood flow in the anterior segment of the eye. *Trans Ophthalmol Soc UK* 1980;**100**:388–97.

Matsui M, Justice J Jr. Anterior segment angiography. In: Justice J Jr, ed. *Ophthalmic Photography*. Boston: Little, Brown and Co; 1982: Chapter 16.

Matsui M, Parel J–M, Weder H, Justice J Jr. Some improved methods of anterior segment fluorescein angiography. *Am J Ophthalmol* 1972;**74**:1075–9.

Meyer PAR, Watson PG. Low dose fluorescein angiography of the conjunctiva and episclera. *Br J Ophthalmol* 1987;**71**:2–10.

Meyer PAR. Patterns of blood flow in episcleral vessels studied by low-dose fluorescein videoangiography. *Eye* 1988;**2**:533–46.

Olver JM, Lee JP. Recovery of anterior segment circulation after strabismus surgery in adult patients. *Ophthalmology* 1992;**99**:305–15.

Ormerod LD *et al*. Anterior segment fluorescein videoangiography with a scanning angiographic microscope. *Ophthalmology* 1990;**97**:745–51.

Talusan ED, Schwartz B. Fluorescein angiography: Demonstration of flow pattern of anterior ciliary arteries. *Arch Ophthamol* 1981;**99**:1074–80.

Watson PG. Anterior segment fluorescein angiography in the surgery of immunologically induced corneal and scleral destructive disorders. *Ophthalmology* 1987;**94**:1452–64.

Watson PG, Bovey E. Anterior segment fluorescein angiography in the diagnosis of scleral inflammation. *Ophthalmology* 1985;**92**:1–11.

Index